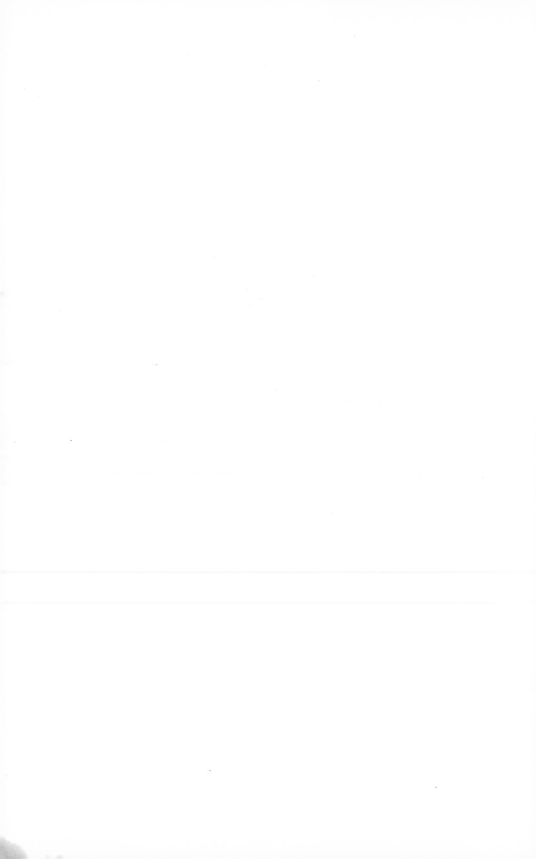

WAR CRIMES IN JAPAN-OCCUPIED INDONESIA

WAR CRIMES
in Japan-Occupied Indonesia

A CASE OF MURDER BY MEDICINE

J. KEVIN BAIRD and SANGKOT MARZUKI

Foreword by MARK HARRISON

Potomac Books
An imprint of the University of Nebraska Press

Library of Congress Cataloging-in-Publication Data

Baird, J. Kevin, author.
War crimes in Japan-occupied Indonesia: a case of murder by medicine / J. Kevin Baird and Sangkot Marzuki;
foreword by Mark Harrison.

pages   cm

Includes bibliographical references and index.

ISBN 978-1-61234-644-1 (cloth: alk. paper)
ISBN 978-1-61234-733-2 (epub)
ISBN 978-1-61234-734-9 (mobi)
ISBN 978-1-61234-645-8 (pdf)
1. Mochtar, Achmad, 1892–1945. 2. World War,
1939–1945—Atrocities—Indonesia. 3. World War,
1939–1945—Atrocities—Japan. 4. Indonesia—
History—Japanese occupation, 1942–1945. 5. War
crimes—Indonesia—History—20th century. 6.
Forced labor—Indonesia—History—20th century. 7.
Tetanus—Vaccination—Indonesia—History—20th
century. 8. Human experimentation in medicine—
Indonesia—History—20th century. I. Marzuki, Sangkot, author. II. Title.
D767.7.B35 2015
940.54'05095982—dc23
2015002823

Set in Scala OT by Lindsey Auten.

In remembrance of the romusha,
their POW brothers, and Iris Chang

CONTENTS

ILLUSTRATIONS

FOREWORD

MARK HARRISON

History is not a science. It is never entirely objective. But historical accounts can be verified or falsified by empirical evidence. When set against the archival record or even the memory of those who witnessed events, some versions of history appear far more plausible than others. Only a handful of die-hard racists would now deny Nazi atrocities and the industrialized slaughter in the death camps, for example. The only real matters for debate in such cases are how many people knew about or willingly participated in these killings. These are questions that cannot easily be answered, but it is important to ask them, and many—including those who inherited the disgusting legacy of Nazi rule—have shown a passionate commitment to the truth. But the same cannot always be said of similar wartime atrocities in Asia. Much of what happened during the Japanese occupation of Asia remains obscure—sometimes deliberately so. There has been reluctance in some quarters to examine allegations and also an attempt to erase the historical record. This began even before the war had ended. We know from American code breakers that on August 15, 1945, the Japanese army was ordered to destroy any potentially incriminating evidence. The next day, a similar order was issued to the navy. Furthermore, on August 24, the Japanese army in Indonesia, and no doubt in other places, was ordered to destroy its caches of chemical weapons and dumdum bullets—articles prohibited by The Hague and Geneva Conventions.

This remarkable book throws a beam of light into a cavern left intentionally dark. J. Kevin Baird and Sangkot Marzuki show how one of Indonesia's most eminent scientists—Professor Achmad Mochtar—

became the scapegoat for a failed experiment that threatened to tarnish the reputation of Indonesia's new rulers, the Japanese. Mochtar was forced to take the blame for the deaths of nine hundred Indonesian laborers (*romusha*) who had been conscripted by the Japanese. The authors make a compelling case that their deaths occurred not through the negligence of Mochtar or even accidental contamination but as a result of a deliberate attempt by the Japanese to poison the *romusha* with tetanus toxin in order to test a weak, improvised vaccine. The unfortunate laborers had been used as human guinea pigs—a fate which befell countless civilians and Allied servicemen who were captured by the Japanese.

Despite efforts at concealment, many of the atrocities committed by the Japanese are known to us, thanks to eyewitness accounts and the diligence of historical researchers. Some of their wartime experiments were attempts to prove the supposed difference or inferiority of other races. Others were the result of wartime expediency—the testing of biological and chemical weapons, experimental vaccines and treatments, and the reactions of the human body to pain and privation. The exploits of Japan's Unit 731 are particularly notorious. Under the command of Dr. Ishii Shiro, the unit's scientists conducted experiments of almost unimaginable cruelty throughout China and other territories seized by the Japanese. It seems that a detachment of this unit may have been operating in Java at the time the lethal vaccinations were administered.

One of the most disturbing things about the events described in this book is that there was no effort to bring the perpetrators to justice. The truth was damaging not only to the Japanese but also to the reputations of Indonesian politicians who had been forced to make difficult compromises with the invaders. Moreover, the volume of cases facing Allied war crimes prosecutors was huge, and some of those responsible for the worst atrocities—like the scientists of Unit 731—were given immunity from prosecution. Some of their findings—such as those relating to the effects of biological and chemical weapons—were potentially useful as tension grew between the West and its communist adversaries. The United States also required the cooperation of Japan in its struggle against communism in the East. As a result, the atrocities committed in Indonesia, China, and many other countries remain unpunished and even unacknowledged. As the authors remark, the Japanese government's failure to accept the full extent of the misery inflicted during the war remains a source of great tension, inflamed recently by the resurgence of Japanese nationalism.

Reading this book, it is easy to become angry at the cruel treatment of Mochtar and thousands of other Indonesians. Indeed, the brutality shown to the romusha by their supposed liberators will come as a revelation to many in the West. And yet the story related here also demonstrates the potential of human beings to rise above ethnic differences. Achmad Mochtar's life bore testimony to this. Despite being an imperial subject, he became the director of one of the world's preeminent institutes of tropical medicine, the Eijkman Institute in Jakarta. This institute—now thriving after its resurrection in 1992—was first established under Dutch rule, but it attracted many foreign researchers and cultivated the talents of Indonesian scientists. It was a site of pioneering research in the fields of deficiency disease and infectious disease, and its work deserves to be more widely known. The institute's achievements are justly celebrated by the authors, who write with passion and insight about an institution which they revere. Sangkot Marzuki is one of Indonesia's most eminent scientists, and he has been director of the Eijkman Institute since it reopened in 1992. Kevin Baird is director of the Eijkman-Oxford Clinical Research Unit, founded in 2007. Their book is an eloquent and moving testimony to a man who remains an inspiration for those who work at the institute and who deserves to be remembered for his intellectual gifts and his humanity. Ultimately, their book is a reminder of the dilemmas we all face as human beings—about our capacity to transform positively or negatively the lives of others.

PREFACE

Our book focuses on a single event during the occupation of Indonesia by Imperial Japan during the Pacific War, the Mochtar affair. Political, historical, and technical elements composed that affair, in which a prominent Indonesian scientist, Achmad Mochtar, signed a coerced confession to mass murder in order to save his colleagues. We strived to gather the available documentary evidence of that event and to present an analysis of known facts aimed at understanding what happened and why. This evidence is carefully detailed, and any gaps are pointed out. We lay out what we consider to be a reasoned estimation of what very likely drove events in the affair. We do so to encourage readers to reach their own conclusions or to bring forth further evidence and analysis, be it conflicting or corroborative.

While we make no pretense of being academic historians applying the fullest rigor of that demanding discipline, we are nonetheless scientists with a deep respect for fact and an engrained aversion to imagination or fantasy in striving to grasp reality. The project represented by this book is thus a work of history by amateur historians. Early in its inception we decided to aim at a broad readership. Key to this decision was the realization that the Mochtar affair was a deeply human drama that occurred within a truly historic period—that is, one rich in events with consequences that reverberate profoundly today in Indonesia and abroad. Mochtar's story reaches across seven decades with its contrast of cruel injustice and deep courage played before the familiar backdrop of the Pacific War and the less familiar drama of the Japanese occupation of Indonesia in that war.

The Mochtar affair hinged upon violent military and political events of this period, 1942 to 1945. That historic context frames Mochtar's story, and in telling it we necessarily convey the history of the birth of the Republic of Indonesia—the fourth most populous nation on earth after China, India, and the United States, and almost certainly the least broadly understood in a cultural and historical sense among those peers. Among Mochtar's friends, family, and colleagues were those who conceived the idea of Indonesia, defined it, and fought to realize it. We strive to express Indonesian national identity because it is essential in understanding the Mochtar affair.

Reaching for an explanation also necessitates engaging the technical complexity of vaccination against tetanus. As our research progressed, this aspect of the Mochtar affair emerged as the most conspicuous weakness in the lies constructed in order to conceal the truth. Prior treatments of this history by nonscientists missed this crucial technical leverage in analyzing Japanese intentions, actions, and deceit. We strive to explain this technical weakness in a lay manner because it underpins the factual deconstruction of the Japanese version of the propaganda that painted Mochtar as a mass murderer.

In short, *War Crimes in Japan-Occupied Indonesia* weaves together complex historical, political, and technical themes in its telling. This synthesis, we believe, conveys the essential truth of what happened to Mochtar. That, in turn, not only restores his dignity, honor, and legacy but also documents the deep heroism he exhibited in forfeiting his life in order to save his colleagues.

At the time of his arrest by the Japanese, Mochtar directed the Eijkman Institute in Jakarta. That institute, with its Nobel Prize heritage, effectively died with the arrest and torture of most of its scientific staff in October 1944 and the execution of Mochtar in July 1945. Though the institute did not formally close until 1965, it had long ceased conducting meaningful medical research. Mochtar's murder, followed immediately by attempted reassertion of colonial domain by Dutch force of arms, destroyed the Eijkman Institute.

We are medical scientists, and we work at that institute today following its resurrection by the government of Indonesia in 1992. Indeed one of us, Sangkot Marzuki, is a successor to Mochtar as director. A portrait of Mochtar hangs at the entrance to Marzuki's suite.

Mochtar is, to us, familiar and omnipresent. His legacy constitutes a key thread of the woven fabric of the institute that lies at the core of our respective professional lives. As many scientists do, we have difficulty segregating our professional and personal passions—they tend to be one and the same. Our science and the institute that permits its expression deeply embeds as a dimension of our respective characters and intellectual beings. The Mochtar affair strikes us very near to the emotional center of a deep wrong committed against a member of our family. We tell his story from that perspective because we cannot be dispassionate. Mochtar's treatment was outrageous, and we do not refrain from expressing heartfelt outrage against it.

The Pacific War is long over, and the Allied victory in that conflict changed the region indelibly and for the better in large and sweeping measures. Formerly belligerent and brutal Japan has since been a peace-loving and positive national presence in the Asian sphere. Japan's rich cultural and intellectual heritage vastly overshadows the cruel fascist darkness it struggles to face and acknowledge as a brief shameful element of its otherwise long and glorious history. Japan's failure to confront its history in that dark period poses a serious threat for humanity in contemporary life. The peoples revering the memories of the victims of that period of Japanese Imperial aggression will not, rightfully, accept anything less than a truthful accounting of their suffering and loss. The people of China, in particular, earned and deserve such. Denial of this right destabilizes Asia and, in economic turn, the world.

Indonesia today is a robust democracy with a thriving economy. This nation and Japan enjoy warm, respectful, and mutually prosperous relationships. Some may rationally see us as callously reopening old and tender wounds connected to the brutal occupation. But we do so with a sense of its necessity. The murder of Achmad Mochtar, and many like him, demands acknowledgment and remembrance. Such justice heals wounds that otherwise fester.

In the case of Indonesia, the occupation left unacknowledged and unredressed injuries without regard to Japan per se. The veiled historic treatment given the brutality visited upon Indonesians simmers within that nation to the present day. The enslavement and murder of at least half a million and perhaps several million young Indonesian men, called romusha, has scarcely been acknowledged by Japan,

Indonesia, or the broader vision of human history. The treatment of the romusha by the occupier and their recruitment, endorsed and promoted by leaders among the occupied, lie at the center of that wound. Most important in the narrow context of the story conveyed in this book, the political character of the romusha program—and its concealed viciousness—effectively drove the events culminating in Mochtar's execution.

In the martyrdom of Mochtar we find both the absolute worst and the very best of the human spirit reflected in the actions of people placed in a hard crucible capable of revealing such. The story offers stark and relevant lessons in being human and having an inborn, assigned, or selected group identity. The selfish pursuit of agendas solely in the better interests of group fellows invites inhumanity to those beyond the group, whereas the pursuit of agendas in the better interests of all invites great humanity. Ideologies and interests tightly constrained to borders of group identity ought to be viewed as intrinsically counter to expression of the best of our humanity. Like individuals, groupings of people may behave selfishly or selflessly. To which of those poles the sum of human communities gravitate very simply defines the quality of the global human experience as dark and miserable or bright and happy. Mochtar's story gives us a clear vision of this dichotomy and the sharp contrast in its expression of the human spirit as wicked or virtuous.

ACKNOWLEDGMENTS

The authors owe many debts of gratitude to friends and colleagues for the assembly of this book. Foremost among those is that owed to Dr. Safarina Malik at the Eijkman Institute. She played a key role in identifying witnesses, approaching them for interviews, and managing those precious sources. Her warm and gracious manner brought us together with those people as likeminded friends rather than simply as sources of information to tap. She reminded us always of the human dimension of this work.

Achmad Mochtar's survivors are among those new friends Dr. Ina brought to us. The recollections and photographs of his nephew and niece, Dr. Asikin Hanafiah and Mrs. Taty Delma Juzar, in Jakarta have deeply enriched this book and our understanding of Mochtar as a man. Discussions with Asikin in particular illuminated this dimension for us with his sharp wit and powerful recall. Mrs. Jolanda van der Bom and her sister, Dr. Monique Hasnah Mochtar (daughters of Imramsyah, son of Mochtar), in Holland very much deepened the history in this book with their photographs and reflections on their late father.

Mrs. Latifah Kodijat Marzoeki in Jakarta (daughter of Dr. Marzoeki and Corrie) generously provided us with documents, photographs, and her extraordinary recollection of the events detailed here. Visiting her home at Tanah Abang, where Marzoeki and Corrie raised her, and hearing her story where it occurred carried the listener to that time. Her gracious generosity in doing so brought an otherwise impossible richness of detail and perspective to the history in this book.

Dr. Ina also found and brought us to Nani Kusumasudjana in Bogor. Nani gives this history its only verbal firsthand accounting of life at the Eijkman Institute during the war and of being held by the Kenpeitai at their prison in Jakarta. We are deeply indebted for her extraordinary courage in revisiting that deep trauma. She cast the sharp light of her recall on otherwise dark corners of the Mochtar affair.

Thanks are also due to Lenny Ekawati and her grandmother, Djumina, for the personal and painful testimony of romusha recruitment practices at one village in Java during the war.

Theodore Friend provided the benefit of his deep knowledge of Indonesia and its history through a long and patient correspondence with us, adding to his already substantial contributions to the historical record on the Mochtar affair. His books, in particular *Blue-Eyed Enemy: Japan against the West in Java and Luzon, 1942–1945* (Princeton University Press, 1988), gave us vital historic facts and perspectives on the colonization and occupation of Indonesia.

We thank Aukje Zuidema and Iris Heidebrink at the Nederlands Instituut voor Oorlogsdocumentatie in Amsterdam (War Archive) for providing us with documentation connected with the Mochtar affair and also for putting us in contact with Jolanda and Monique. Their own book, *Encyclopedia of Indonesia in the Pacific War* (Brill, 2010), served as a rich source of material concerning the Japanese occupation.

Vera Chrisverani and Lies Rahayu Dwi labored with us over the four years of putting this book together, helping us to manage manuscripts, materials, correspondence, and appointments around our busy schedules. Byron Laursen provided editing and valued suggestions on composition. Our editors at the University of Nebraska Press, Bridget Barry and Sabrina Ehmke-Sergeant, worked with extraordinary patience with us, and we are grateful to them for that and the mentoring in publishing done along the way.

Finally, our literary agent, Ann Collette at the Rees Agency of Boston, embraced this project with a sincere passion for the humanity of the tale. She coached, cajoled, and reminded us of the importance of having Mochtar's story become more widely known.

Acknowledgments

WAR CRIMES IN JAPAN-OCCUPIED INDONESIA

ONE

Calamity

In the Life Span of a Maize Plant

The island of Java lies between Sumatra and Bali in the tropical seas of Southeast Asia. It is the social, political, and economic fulcrum of modern Indonesia's 245 million people, their hundreds of distinct languages, and dizzying array of cultures scattered across 13,500 islands astride the equator. The Republic of Indonesia has a land area approximating that of Western Europe stretching across 3,300 miles—a span as far as San Francisco to Bermuda, or from London to Kabul. Java alone has the same land area as Greece, with twelve times the population. The archipelago boasts enormous biological diversity, staggering mineral and agricultural wealth, and an astonishingly rich human history.

A thousand years ago, a constellation of sophisticated Hindu kingdoms dotted the island of Java. From 1135 to 1157, the well-loved King Joyoboyo reigned over a prosperous era in the kingdom of Kediri, in eastern Java. Joyoboyo reunited this divided kingdom, and the time of his rule was a golden age in Javanese literature. But his greatest mark on the history and culture of Java actually came in the years following his stepping down from the throne to pursue spiritual enlightenment. The profound and indelible Joyoboyo legacy lingers today, after almost a full millennium, and it resonated with eerie power in the years surrounding World War II.

Living as a mystic recluse after his abdication, Joyoboyo—thought by some to be an incarnation of the Hindu god Vishnu—wrote lengthy poetic epics filled with stirring prophecies. One of them, *Pralembang*

Joyoboyo, foretold that the people of Java would be ruled for three centuries by white people, and then, for the life span of a maize plant, by yellow dwarfs from the northeast. Next would come the return of the Ratu Adil, the Just King. When iron wagons could drive without horses and when ships could sail through the sky, he predicted, the Ratu Adil would arrive. Then the Javanese would again rule their own lands. This prophecy played a hand in the unfolding of the history conveyed in this book.

In 1941 the people of Indonesia had endured more than three centuries of Dutch colonial rule. First came the avaricious Dutch East Indies Company, the VOC, and later the Dutch Crown government. Each indulged in massive exploitation of Indonesia's abundance of natural resources, including the sweat and labor of generations of Indonesians held in indentured servitude. Consistent with the Javanese belief in history as cyclic, people began to sense at the dawn of the 1940s that their deliverance was at hand. Three hundred and twenty-two years had passed since the 1619 establishment of a VOC post at Jaya Karta on the north coast of western Java. The Dutch would rename the city Batavia. It would be renamed Djakarta after the Dutch defeat in 1942, and finally it became Jakarta when Dutch phonetics were abandoned in 1950. In accordance with Joyoboyo, the Javanese of 1941 believed that this long period of foreign domination would soon end.

The Dutch in the Netherlands East Indies of 1941 had anxiously watched from afar as the Nazi jackboot heel crushed freedom in Europe, including the invasion and occupation of their homeland. The Nazi–Imperial Japanese axis, though, seemed a nearly irrelevant political abstraction. The Japanese invasion of China, which had begun a decade earlier, remained a distant ugliness not impacting their comfortable lives in the East Indies. The Dutch colonialists scarcely imagined the events in China as a prelude to their eviction by Imperial Japan. Japan's military was not perceived as a threat: feeling secure in their East Indies stronghold, the Dutch colonialists had held fund-raisers to support the war effort in Europe rather than for their own defense.

The colonized peoples of Netherlands East Indies watched these events from a wholly different perspective. Joyoboyo's "yellow dwarfs" from the northeast appeared poised to challenge the three-century reign of whites over Java and much of Asia. In January 1941, Mohammad Husni Thamrin, leader of a nascent nationalist movement, cited Joyoboyo's hope-stirring prophecies in this context in a public speech. Dutch authorities placed him under house arrest for doing so, under suspicion that the drawing of such a connection between prophecy and reality constituted sympathy with the Japanese. Already ill, Thamrin died a few days later. He is considered a great early hero of the Indonesian Republic, and a major thoroughfare in contemporary Jakarta bears his name.

The events of December 7 and 8, 1941, filled the deeply mystical Javanese with enormous hope and wonder. First, the Imperial Japanese struck their incredibly forceful and devastating blow at Pearl Harbor. Then, without pause, they pivoted their military might to seize all of Southeast Asia in an audacious single broad stroke. Suddenly Indonesia's long-held dream of independence seemed to be flowing from the pages of *Pralembang Joyoboyo* to the pages of history. If they could tolerate the occupation of the Japanese for what was essentially a few seconds in the larger sweep of history, soon their Just King would rise. Steel wagons without horses and ships sailing through the air, bearing the Rising Sun of Imperial Japan, had been unleashed upon the white colonialists of Asia. Indonesians welcomed this invader as a liberator and acted in anticipation of a hasty exit resulting in their freedom and independence.

The Japanese occupiers—who with relative ease took all of Indonesia by early April 1942—would come to understand that Joyoboyo's prophecy was widely credited in this newly subjugated territory. The occupation forces worried a great deal, though, about interpretation of the corn cycle in Joyoboyo's writings and the brevity expected of their rule. The Kenpeitai, Japan's notorious equivalent of Hitler's ss, closely interrogated Indonesian scholars on its meaning. One of them, Slamet Imam Santoso, played phonetic sleight of hand with the Javanese words, substituting *praja agung* (great kingdom) for *jagung* (corn), thereby placating the Japanese with the idea that Joyoboyo had predicted the yellow man would stay in power as long as the kingdom was great.[1] And the Japanese privately believed, in the first flush of their conquest, they would be masters of Indonesia for eons to come.

For a decade prior to the invasion, militarists had controlled Japan's government and infused that nation with a spirit of conquest and domination bent upon elevating the Japanese as the ruling masters of all of Asia, much in the model of Hitler's "Thousand Year Third Reich" for all of Europe. The Imperial Japanese shared the racist and fascist worldview of the Nazis and allied to that cruel cause. The invading armies representing those masters also believed that such a destiny was theirs to grasp in the name of the emperor of Japan. Though they duplicitously spoke of a free Indonesia, they acted precisely as what they were, colonial imperialists. They planned for the colonial mastery of the East Indies with victory in the Pacific War they had engineered to those ends.

Like their Nazi friends, the Imperial Japanese were hugely mistaken. *Pralembang Joyoboyo* played out as expressed, although Joyoboyo did not foretell of the brutality to be endured in that short span of time. Japanese mastery of Indonesia eventually echoed the famous phrase that seventeenth-century English philosopher Thomas Hobbes used to describe the lives of early humans: it was nasty, brutish, and short.

In that limited time, lasting only the forty months from March 1942 until August 1945, several million Indonesians—no one knows the total number—lost their lives at the hands of this new foreign occupier. None of these dead fought in pitched battle or carried a weapon of any kind. They all died in a Japanese custody cynically veiled in a deeply insincere fraternal regard for Indonesian nationalist aspirations.

Romusha

The majority of these stunning losses occurred through the recruitment or, more often, impressment of young Indonesian men from Java into a highly organized corps of laborers. These *romusha* (a Japanese word for coolie or unskilled laborer adopted into Indonesian language as a term for a slave laborer) were collected from thousands of villages across Java. These collections were conducted with the cooperation of local authorities at the behest of nationalist leadership. Working in cause for the victory of Japan was promoted as working in cause for the freedom and independence of Indonesia.

These romusha traveled by train to railheads near ports on Java, where they were held in guarded camps prior to transport by ship to distant worksites. By almost all accounts, they were taken to mines, plantations, and sites of construction of military roads, rails, bridges, and airfields all through the Indonesian archipelago and beyond. They indeed worked in cause of Imperial Japanese military dominance of the region and, in so doing, the defeat of the western colonial imperialists. Superficially at least, the labor represented a win-win for the occupier and occupied.

In reality, however, the romusha were being systematically killed. Once effectively out of sight of the collaborating Indonesian political elites who mobilized them, they faced confinement and harsh physical treatment similar to that meted out to Allied prisoners of war—starvation, backbreaking labor, beatings, and summary executions. Of the estimated 4 to 10 million men taken into captivity in this way, several million were unaccounted for and presumed dead.

This is a stunning indictment for several reasons. Some are complex but rationally explainable, while others are plainly baffling. Most readers of this book will have had no inkling of the scale of murder of the romusha by the Japanese. The reasons for this are explained through the course of this book. What evades explanation here or elsewhere is the sheer brutality the Japanese directed toward people working in direct support of their war effort. At best, the Japanese lacked the resources to make their labor projects humane and survivable, and the romusha were simply worked to death. At worst, the Japanese labored to whittle down the manpower available to confront them when their imperial colonial designs later became obvious to occupied nations. The evidence from dozens of work sites across Southeast Asia all point to one inescapable truth—the Japanese willfully killed these men both obliquely by completely neglecting their most basic human needs and directly by beatings and summary executions. We cannot know what drove them to do so.

Reliable death rates for romusha at projects within Indonesia are exceptional. Documentation of their movements and repatriation rarely occurred. However, about 280,000 romusha were documented as exported from Java, and only 52,000 were subsequently documented as repatriated after the war.[2] Survival rates ranging between 20 to 50 percent may be considered plausible and perhaps typical. Death rates for romusha involved in construction of the Burma-Thailand railway, for example, were compared to POWs by Lt. Col. William A. Henderson: "Approximately 27 percent of the Allied soldiers and almost 50 percent of the Southeast Asian impressed laborers died working on the railroad."[3] Dr. Robert Hardie, interred near that rail project, described the hellish conditions: "We hear of the frightful casualties from cholera and other diseases among these people and of the brutality with which they are treated by the Japanese. People who have been near the camps speak with bated breath of the state of affairs—corpses rotting unburied in the jungle, almost complete lack of sanitation, frightful stench, overcrowding, swarms of flies. There is no medical attention in these camps, and the wretched natives are of course unable to organise any communal sanitation."[4] Likewise, an Australian POW surgeon on the Thai-Burma road project recorded, "Endless streams of wretched Coolies from Malaya are plodding their slippery way to the jungle road. Those who speak English frequently have sad words to say about the recruiting methods the Nipponese used to secure their services. These poor wretches are dying up here in countless thousands."[5] Among the many dead were those summarily executed for having faltered at the wrong moment, showed defiance, stolen some morsel of food, or tried to flee the hell of that captivity.

The murder of several million young Indonesian romusha is perhaps the least known of holocausts visited upon noncombatants in World War II. Its horrors were effectively buried by postwar political exigencies in the new Republic of Indonesia and the region. Those will be detailed later in this book. The plight of the romusha, and their veiled treatment in history, remains a politically charged issue in contemporary Indonesia.

The Japanese carefully concealed the lethal viciousness of the program with humane treatment of the romusha when within sight of Indonesian political leaders and their base of 50 million people on Java. The cooperation on romusha sustained good relations between the leaders of the occupier and occupied. The accidental murder of 900 romusha by a Japanese medical experiment at a transit camp on the outskirts of Jakarta in 1944 was the defining event of the Mochtar affair. It politically rippled widely and dangerously for the Japanese. They would conjure saboteurs to mitigate those consequences.

Conspirators, Spies, and Saboteurs

The suffering of the romusha "volunteers" enlisted in supporting Japan's war efforts emphasizes the extreme degree of brutality that the occupiers were capable of directing toward people whom they perceived as actually hostile and threatening to their empire. Many thousands of these real or imagined enemies were summarily executed, or when suspicion rather than mere convenience motivated the Japanese, torture would come first. Many others were subjected to martial legal proceedings, formally condemned, and finally executed.

Many of these victims fit a profile of persecution by the Japanese. They often possessed lands and wealth that Imperial Japan desired, or they were local or regional leaders under the Dutch, spoke a European language, or had been educated in Europe. Ethnic Chinese and Eurasians were favored targets, as were intellectuals of any race or creed.

A particularly egregious example of the capricious nature of these murders is the massacre of more than 21,000 people at Pontianak in West Borneo between April 1943 and June 1944. The victims included noblemen, doctors, academics, business leaders, and ordinary citizens apparently chosen at random.[6] At the war tribunal hearings of the Japanese officers responsible for these massacres, it emerged that they had concocted the alleged China-inspired rebellion cited as justifying the murders. They had conspired to improve their opportunities for promotion by cruelly and efficiently quelling a nonexistent rebellion. The perceived scale of threat of the rebellion, they reasoned, would be proportionate to the number of people they executed. That number, in turn, correlated to the scale of their service to the empire and their subsequent likelihood of promotion.

The stories of individual murders and their rippling consequences to families and the nation are buried in the numbingly vast numbers of Indonesians subjected to inhumane labor, starvation, torture, and murder. Among these murders, the circumstances and consequences of one in particular are at least reasonably well documented.

As his titles imply, Professor Doctor Achmad Mochtar was a person of great learning, one of the brightest lights of medicine and science in the nascent Indonesian nation. He hailed from the intellectually proud Minangkabau people of western Sumatra and was a devoted husband and father of two sons. In casual photographs taken immediately before the war—when Mochtar was approaching fifty—his smile conveys pride and happiness, and his eyes shine with the confidence of an accomplished man who was well traveled, well read, and successfully engaged in deeply meaningful and intellectually challenging humanitarian work within a highly prestigious institute of medical research.

In an act of political desperation, the Imperial Japanese deceitfully cast Mochtar as a remotely plausible scapegoat for what we surmise was a criminal medical experiment of their own design that had gone terribly wrong. The Japanese experiment and its outcome not only threatened the illusion of their beneficence for Indonesians but also led to the fates of the actual perpetrators of that experiment— wearing the uniforms of the Imperial Japanese Army—who would, if they could not deflect the blame, face war tribunal justice. Their diabolical use of Mochtar protected their occupation and, at its end, their personal liberty.

In stark contrast to the cruelty and cowardice of his accusers, Mochtar's response to their duplicity shines as the finest noble potential of the human spirit. He willingly sacrificed himself to save his colleagues.

An Execution

Late in the afternoon of July 3, 1945, it may be surmised that two Japanese sentries would have escorted Indonesia's finest native-born scientist and physician to his ritual meeting with the executioner's sword. Mochtar had been slender in his normal life. After ten months of imprisonment, the first three under severe torture, he undoubtedly would have been rail-thin and feeble. A dirty cotton sack would have covered his head, a ritual for those condemned by the Imperial Japanese.

This would have been a walk the guards had already made hundreds of times in past weeks, months, and years with other condemned prisoners. It was their routine—another day at the office.

Perhaps they smoked cigarettes and chatted amicably as they gripped Mochtar's withered arms above the elbows. His hands would have been bound behind him. They would have allowed his weak steps to set their leisurely pace over the hundred yards or so between the truck that transported him from the jail and a bloodstained patch of mud near a large scraggly tree that stood near the Java Sea at an isolated marsh on Jakarta's waterfront.

Having properly positioned Mochtar, they would have removed the sack, replacing it with a blindfold, exposing the back of Mochtar's neck so the executioner's blow might more accurately hit its mark. The efficacy of the executioner's sword stroke—by Imperial Japanese lights, the most aesthetically correct way to kill and to die—might be spoiled if the victim were to see the long, well-polished blade arcing overhead and to instinctively recoil.

Mochtar would not yet have been certain of the purpose of his transport from the jail on that day. He probably began to understand as they approached the killing ground—the stench of death at this place would have been overpowering. Certainly with the placement of the blindfold and seeing the remote surroundings and his executioners, Mochtar would know the end was nigh.

Before the blindfold had been placed, Mochtar perhaps caught a final glimpse of this world. The sun at that hour on that date would have been poised low to his left in clear sky above the Java Sea facing him, setting it ablaze with ochre yellows, oranges, and reds. He surely thought of his beloved wife, Siti Hasnah, their two boys, and what had been their superbly rich life together. He may have mused at his rise from village boy in remote Sumatra to country doctor to head of the world's leading scientific institute for tropical medicine. He would not live to see the emergence of a free and sovereign Indonesia, but among his friends, colleagues, and relations were many of the architects of that achievement. He knew before his arrest that the Americans were bearing down hard on Imperial Japan, and he would have known that his murderers were also doomed.

Mochtar would also have known why he was being murdered—to protect the Japanese murderers of hundreds of young Indonesian men. His rage would be tempered by the inner grace of having saved many of his colleagues from this horrific fate.

A nearby officer would have nodded, and the waiting swordsman standing behind Mochtar would have barked an order as he drew his weapon to the ready. The sentry would have pushed Mochtar to his knees, then backed away, absently flicking his cigarette stub into the crimson mud. The executioner would have lifted his sword high overhead with both hands, then with all possible force sliced through Mochtar's neck, pairing the stroke with a constricted, guttural shout. His murderers would have waited for the flow of blood to abate, then picked up his head and dragged his body to a foul mound of earth nearby. The sentries would have shoveled dirt over his remains to mitigate the stench of rot that had pervaded this awful patch of earth for more than three years.

By the time Achmad Mochtar's life ended beside that forlorn tree near the water's edge, Imperial Japan was itself being driven to its knees by relentless American armed forces. The Pacific War would be over in six short weeks. But political expediencies that would outlast the war ensured both Mochtar's doom and the almost equally heartless ruin of his reputation and legacy.

Understanding his terrifying journey requires us, more than half a century later, to dismantle the false accusations that protected his murderers and to overcome the loss of key evidence that was either physically destroyed or buried in Japanese-language archives inaccessible to most of us. It forces us to understand the complex and nuanced Japanese motivations for murdering an innocent, valuable, highly principled man just before they lost their brief hold on Indonesia. But by peeling back the time-crusted lies and clearing away the fog of war, we find a story of incredible devotion and sacrifice, an amazing counterpoint to the murderous brutality of a dark era. We then meet in Mochtar's story a great, unsung hero of the Pacific War and of a nation that emerged from its turmoil, the Republic of Indonesia.

Useful and Ugly Racism

For centuries, native peoples throughout Southeast Asia had resented the European colonial domination of their homelands. Only Siam, now known as Thailand, had escaped subjugation, thanks to shrewd diplomatic concessions with Britain and internal government reforms creating a constitutional monarchy (Democracy Monument standing today in old Bangkok was erected in 1939). Vietnam and Cambodia were French Indochina, the English ruled Burma and the Federated Malay States, and American domination of the Philippines came around 1900 at the end of centuries of Spanish reign. These colonial powers effectively managed the civil and legal affairs, security, and wealth of the millions of indigenous Southeast Asian peoples.

The ruthless military clique that held sway in independent Tokyo in the 1930s did not so much resent those foreign presences as deeply envy them. They saw East Asia as their property to seize and manage. They conceived the Greater East Asia Co-Prosperity Sphere as propaganda aiding in the military wresting of control from those western colonial powers. It put Imperial Japan in the ruling position—a nakedly self-interested ambition that they cloaked by cynically exploiting their racial proximity to the peoples whose lands they conquered and by holding out false hopes of pathways to independence. An elaborate political dance with emerging leaders of the nascent Indonesian nation was a key Japanese ploy for keeping those illusory hopes glimmering, and that delicate dance of power and fear demanded Mochtar's martyrdom.

The hubris of the Japanese conquerors exceeded even that of the western colonialists. Few races in this era held their supremacy as high or as earnestly as the Imperial Japanese. Like their Aryan Nazi friends in the European sphere, they perceived the lives of the races they had conquered as valueless and disposable. The evidence of fact on this is concrete, but some Japanese today wish it away and insist that their countrymen fought nobly with the intent of liberating East Asia from the colonial imperialism of their "blue-eyed" enemies. In reality the Japanese armed forces conducted wholesale enslavement, murder, and rape of the peoples they had "liberated" with the sole intent of establishing dominion over them. As one Japanese general exhorted his troops on the eve of the invasion of colonial Southeast Asia, "With one blow you will annihilate the blue-eyed enemy and their black slaves." Theodore Friend explained, "Japanese militant enthusiasm fed on racial feeling to strengthen it for defeat of Americans and Dutch, and for subjugation of Filipinos and Indonesians. . . . No clearer fighting distinction between 'us' and 'them' could be drawn."[7] The Japanese likely viewed their new wards more as "black slaves" than as fellow Asians.

The simple notion of racial superiority, as tragically taught in human history again and again, imbues the "superior" with a misplaced moral liberty to enslave and slaughter the "inferior." The Imperial Japanese of the Pacific War added yet another wretched chapter to that history.

The racial, national, and criminal ugliness visited upon the occupied peoples of Asia during the Pacific War continue to reverberate across the region. Northeast Asia today is a political and military tinderbox in large measure because of the brutality of Japan's domination of the region seventy years ago. In 2012 enraged mobs in Chinese cities destroyed Japanese property and products over a territorial dispute involving barren, rocky islands with some seabed resources. The disputed territory itself does not incite such passions. China's indelible national memory of Imperial Japanese hauteur and inhumanity, along with their reasoned perception of Japan's failure to acknowledge those wrongs, does.

Denial and Dishonor

Many influential groups in modern Japan present the nation as a victim of the Pacific War. They hold the destruction of Japan's cities and many of its residents as the result of unprovoked aggression and cruelty. The armed forces of Imperial Japan, these groups assert, had been crushed in their righteous war against colonial imperialism in Asia. The Yasukuni Shrine in Tokyo memorializes the Japanese soldiers and sailors lost in the wars of 1867–1951, and its museum expresses explicitly that these men surrendered their lives in the Pacific War in heroic self-defense of the Japanese motherland against European Imperialism.[8] This somehow gives a pass to those responsible for most of the losses: the Americans. The naked militaristic aggression and monstrous behavior of its armed forces during that war—for which many national leaders, officers, and men were tried, convicted, and executed or imprisoned—is not widely credited in Japan. In October 2006 Japanese Prime Minister Shinzo Abe, for example, asserted that the men convicted by the Allied tribunals "are not war criminals under the laws of Japan."[9]

When senior Japanese government officers pay their respects at Yasukuni (as Prime Minister Abe did on December 26, 2013), they provoke the anger of the formerly occupied nations. Implicit in such homage is rejection of the responsibility for crimes against humanity and the validity of the justice meted out. The official homage paid at Yasukuni serves to affirm the historically preposterous notion of noble martyrdom suffered by Imperial Japan's military in the Pacific War. The website for Yasukuni explains that the honored include those "who were labeled war criminals and executed after having been tried by the Allies." Most dictionaries of English define the word *labeled* as "a classifying phrase or name applied to a person or thing, especially one that is inaccurate." The website states that "divinities enshrined at Yasukuni Shrine all sacrificed their lives to the public duty of protecting their motherland."[10] Abe said of his 2013 visit to the shrine, "I prayed to pay respect for the war dead who sacrificed their precious lives." The formerly occupied nations of East Asia—and the former colonial powers—may well wonder how they threatened the Japanese homeland in the 1930s and early 1940s, and why so many of their unarmed citizens lost their own precious lives. The Imperial Japanese military men indeed sacrificed themselves, but not before sacrificing many others in the cause of the enrichment and elevation of their race.

Try to imagine the reaction among European neighbors if a German chancellor were to solemnly visit a shrine in Berlin honoring the memories and sacrifices made by men like Himmler, Göring, Hitler, and their henchmen. Such a visit would be rationally construed as honoring the Nazis as patriotic martyrs of Allied aggression and unjust vengeance against them. It would also be acknowledged as a grotesque affront to millions of their victims. No such monument could possibly exist in modern Germany because that nation has accepted the truth of the Nazis' inhumanity. The German nation chooses to honor the victims. German chancellors visit the sites of Nazi atrocities and pay homage to those slaughtered. This sort of justice permits sincere forgiveness and healing. Japanese actions in contemporary life instead invite fury and deepened injury among the formerly occupied and brutalized nations.

Chinese Foreign Ministry spokesman Qin Gang issued this statement in response to Abe's 2013 visit to the Yasukuni Shrine: "We strongly protest and condemn the Japanese leader's acts." He called the visits "an effort to glorify the Japanese militaristic history of external invasion and colonial rule . . . and to challenge the outcome of World War II." The unequivocal outrage expressed by the government of China, supported by the known facts of the Pacific War, finds voice with no other globally influential government. Indifference to Japanese revision of this history amounts to a cold indifference to those murdered by them. In a moral sense, China stands virtually alone on the right side of history regarding Japan's systematic perversion of what actually occurred in the Pacific War.

The U.S. government, in contrast, seems loath to challenge or upset its key strategic partner, especially in the context of a geopolitical contest with a rising regional competitor. The U.S. embassy in Tokyo issued the following statement on December 26, 2013, in response to Abe's visit to Yasukuni: "Japan is a valued ally and friend. Nevertheless, the United States is disappointed that Japan's leadership has taken an action that will exacerbate tensions with Japan's neighbors."[11] This mild rebuke made headline news, if for no other reason than the extreme rarity of such on this topic from U.S. officialdom. The statement expresses no disagreement with the spirit of the visit to Yasukuni, only regret at its consequences. Taken at face value, it is a morally hollow response steeped in strategic interests. That sentiment should provoke deep worry for both the stability of a volatile and vitally important region and the moral standing of the government expressing it.

We cannot imagine the U.S. government today describing any nation honoring the Nazis as revered martyrs as its "valued ally and friend." Even less so would it tacitly accept that view by completely failing to challenge it. That would amount to accepting denial of Nazi responsibility for the Jewish holocaust throughout Europe. How does the Japanese government's reverence for the men responsible for the frank murder of at least as many Asians not evoke the same moral stance? Compelling geopolitics effaces moral clarity on painful truths bearing high strategic costs in their honest management. Another truth is that the failure of such honesty eventually bears very heavy costs.

Today China challenges the decades-long stabilizing presence of the U.S. Navy and strong American alliances in East Asia. China's rigid and muscular posture on questionable and aggressive maritime claims provokes judicious anxiety and consternation among its neighbors. The hope for peaceful resolution of these disputes among the contestants would perhaps be more likely realized by first resolving a powerful moral conflict regarding the truth of a crucial shared history. China facing rivals in denial of that history steels its moral certitude and national resolve against them.

The Japanese view of their invasion and occupation of China and the region as a noble defense of their homeland against white colonial imperialists finds unequivocal expression in the deep reverence for the memories of the men responsible for the brutality that occurred. Honoring the Imperial Japanese military as national martyrs rejects their direct responsibility for the frank murder of millions of noncombatants. That rejection, in turn, overtly dishonors their victims and incites genuine fury in those who bore their loss. It is a grave injustice.

Swimming with Sharks

Western readers probably know about the terrible suffering and heroism of Allied soldiers who fought and died on obscure, remote islands like Guadalcanal, Eniwetok Atoll, Tarawa, Wakde, Biak, Saipan, and Iwo Jima. These military men and women served the liberty of humanity honorably and nobly in confronting a racist and fascist enemy. They also suffered as prisoners in such atrocities as the Bataan Death March and the slow annihilation of thousands of British, Australian, and Dutch prisoners of war at the camp at Sandakan, Borneo. The bloody battle for China dragged on for fourteen cruel and costly years. The military confrontation in the Pacific War carried unprecedented combat ferocity, mercilessness, and underlying racial hatreds.

Allied soldiers faced their Japanese foes more or less as equals, each pitted against the destruction of the other by force of arms. The unarmed civilians facing the Japanese military in their occupied homelands had a different experience and a far more terrifying one. Death or torture of Indonesian civilians at the hands of the

Japanese occupier often came swiftly, unexpectedly, and incomprehensibly. People carried on with their lives as the Japanese around them went about the business of stripping away anything of value or belligerently countering real, imagined, or conjured threats to their occupation. This was not combat, but it was a war nonetheless punctuated by a clear and present danger of losing one's life or liberty. The illusion of normalcy deepened the terror.

A man could be pulled from his home or office, jailed, tortured, and beheaded simply because he was rich, spoke a European language, or was considered highly educated. The logic of such events hinged upon inscrutable and often shifting rationales. The Japanese concocted plots and conspiracies against their occupation to achieve, by ordinary Indonesian civilian lights, undeclared and utterly unknown aims. To the innocents who were swept up in their stratagems, the killings often appeared as simply random murder.

Although some of the populace appeared especially vulnerable, no one was immune. The experience of the occupied peoples of Asia may be compared to that of people adrift in shark-infested waters. The sharks may attack. Or they may not. Dorsal fins split the surface, and shadows are seen approaching and then passing. The military occupation government's willingness to attack whomever, whenever, and wherever they wanted was unpredictable and thus impossible to avoid. The sharks prowled the waters of occupation by their own unknowable impulses and instincts.

What provoked the Japanese to murder civilians in occupied Netherlands East Indies was often simply an idea, one of their own rather than of their victims. They distrusted "half-breed" Eurasians—anathema to their closely held notions of racial purity and order—no matter their political leanings. Chinese Indonesians were, by Imperial Japanese lights, genetically untrustworthy. Like all governments suffering the poison of fascism, the Japanese feared intellectuals of any race or creed, and they too suffered severely. The occupiers coveted the riches of the wealthy and often framed them within conjured conspiracies in order to seize that wealth by legal deceits.

Members of these groups were more exposed to risk of sudden execution than others. Indonesians who looked Eurasian or Chinese, spoke Dutch, had a higher education, or owned nice things was in effect treading those shark-filled waters while injured and bleeding. They were more likely to trigger the murderous instincts of the sharks. But—and this added to the terror—neither these "liabilities" nor their absence was any guarantee of being either consumed or safe. Each person could only carry on, waking up each day, going to work or on family outings, all the time wondering if this was the day the Imperial Japanese shark would take him or her down.

Prof. Dr. Achmad Mochtar was reasonably wealthy. He had been educated extensively, both in Indonesia and in Holland. He spoke fluent Dutch. A scientific paper he had published before the war disproved the flawed research of an extremely prominent Japanese scientist, making Mochtar vulnerable to the charge of being anti-Japanese. In these regards, he had been a likely target from day one of the occupation. But he was also very highly respected and connected with powerful Indonesian political elites. The Japanese were careful to create the impression that they nurtured Indonesia's nationalist ambitions, positioning themselves as big brothers who would ultimately guide their little brothers into self-sufficiency. Mochtar, as both the director of a medical research institute and vice rector of a school of medicine, had degrees of protection.

But a day came when the Japanese needed him to be guilty of a crime they had committed. So the Kenpeitai took him away, tortured him along with his fellow scientists, extracted a false confession, and later, just as the Allies closed in, killed him. The most shocking aspect of Mochtar's execution, and that of the nine hundred romusha he was accused of murdering, is that the men who perpetrated these crimes actually got away with them.

Wholesale Justice

The Pacific War cost the lives of millions of Koreans, Chinese, Vietnamese, Cambodians, Lao, Thai, Burmese, Malaysians, Indonesians, Filipinos, Papuans, and others. It also claimed many tens of thousands of Europeans, Americans, and Australians. With the exception of the Americans, the majority of these people were noncombatants: resident alien and indigenous civilians alike and prisoners of war. The militarists in Tokyo of the 1930s plotted and carried out this war, citing only their frustration in obtaining the strategic commodities for gaining military dominance as justification for that warfare.

After Japan's surrender, the Allies meted out some justice for these crimes. Trials of twenty-eight Japanese leaders resulted in seven death sentences, sixteen life sentences, two terms of imprisonment (seven and twenty years), the deaths of two prisoners before being sentenced, and, in the case of Okawa Shumei, former director of the East Asiatic Economic Investigation Bureau, dismissal with a successful plea of insanity. Among the officers and men of the Imperial Japanese armed forces, 5,700 were tried for war crimes, resulting in 984 death sentences, 475 life imprisonments, 2,944 finite prison terms, 1,018 acquittals, and 279 cases with outcomes such as insanity, death in prison, or dismissal of charges.[12] Those executed are among the men honored at the Yasukuni Shrine, along with the many who evaded justice for their crimes by not surviving the war.

Many criminals among the Japanese survivors of the Pacific War also escaped justice. The net cast by war tribunals for these sharks could only be described as large gauge, and many swam through it effortlessly. The Allies gave highest priority to crimes against prisoners of war. While being arraigned before the Australian military tribunal for the murder of fifteen Indonesians in a medical experiment, Navy surgeon Captain Nakamura Hirosato entered into evidence the following news clipping from the United Press:

Australia to Liberate Nippon War Suspects
Sydney, Feb. 10

The *Sydney Sun* in a dispatch from Tokyo Tuesday said "at least 90 percent of Japanese war criminal suspects charged with murder, torture, and other atrocities in New Guinea and New Britain will be freed on February 20."

The *Sun* said, "The Australian Government ordered the release of these men because their crimes were not committed against Australian servicemen but only against Australian civilians (mainly plantation managers) and American and British and Dutch civilians, missionaries, and courageous natives who helped save the lives of Australian and American servicemen."

The *Sun* said, "For reasons unknown . . . Canberra ruled only those Japanese charged with offenses against Australian service personnel will be tried."[13]

The "reasons unknown" will be revisited at the closing of this history. In 1951 the Cold War raged. The United States discovered new friends in former enemies and new enemies in former friends. New geopolitical pragmatism skewed moral stances so far as old war crimes were concerned. All Japanese war criminals still in prison in 1958 were released on the grounds of fine points of evidentiary process during the war tribunals, such as permitting entry of hearsay evidence. Many in Japan accepted that outcome as legal vindication of their conduct of the Pacific War.

At Manus Island in 1951, Nakamura's defense counsel rationally argued that the military tribunal had exceeded its remit in seeking to prosecute his client for the murder of Indonesian nationals. In other words, he contended that higher authorities considered the murders of innocent civilians not significant enough to be pursued. The wide gaps in the net cast by Allied prosecutors, as reported in the news article, indeed implied this to be true, but the tribunal rejected the argument, and Nakamura's case went to trial. The courtroom transcripts of that trial provide key insights that help illuminate the Mochtar affair and will be considered in detail in chapter 11.

Murder by Medicine

There were many conspicuously heinous murderers who escaped justice of any kind. Most notable of these may be Ishii Shiro and the notorious Unit 731 he commanded. This "unit" was actually a vast network of military biological research assets, including activities for both medical advancement (drugs, vaccines, preventive medicine, and hygiene) and the development of biological weaponry. The unit effectively harnessed many thousands of Japan's best and brightest medical and scientific minds. Their work under the command of Ishii was conducted throughout the Japanese Empire: China, Taiwan, the Philippines, Singapore, and Indonesia. Whether in pursuit of medical or biological warfare objectives, the experimentation methods under Ishii's leadership were immoral by any standard and often macabre and sadistic as well. Documentation exists of dissections of conscious prisoners who were not anaesthetized, including American POWs in Japan and China—the scientists wished to know that anesthesia did not impact surgical outcomes or the course of induced infections surgically observed.

The astonishing cruelty of these men of medicine seemed to know no bounds. In China they tied healthy prisoners to posts spread out over a wide geographic area and then carefully measured the efficacy of various release methods for diseases like anthrax and plague. A similar approach was taken to measure the kill radius of explosives. In one whimsical experiment, the doctors amputated the arms of a prisoner and attempted to reattach them on opposite sides. Starving Chinese children in villages were visited by Japanese scientists bearing sweet rolls carrying the germs of cholera or typhoid in tests of the virulence of those bacterial strains. Unit 731 airplanes dropped canisters of plague-carrying fleas onto uncontested Chinese cities—and to the present day endemic plague still occurs in those once plague-free areas. The unit occasionally enlisted the aid of local Kenpeitai to kidnap ordinary citizens of occupied territories off the streets when the supply of prisoners to fill the rosters of their experiments ran low.[14]

The work of Unit 731 lacked the slightest concern for the excruciating suffering and terrifying deaths of their many thousands of test subjects—men, women, children, and infants. In terms of numbers of victims and cruelty of methods, the Japanese scientists vastly exceeded their Nazi counterparts at work in European concentration camps. Unlike those Nazi doctors who were assiduously pursued and executed, the Japanese scientists completely escaped being brought to justice, including their commander, Ishii Shiro. None were arrested, much less jailed or arraigned for trial.

The U.S. government, to its lasting and deep shame, not only granted the key players of Unit 731 immunity from prosecution but also paid substantial cash sums in exchange for the data collected by their systematic and astonishingly cruel murders. The data on biological weaponry and its effects, impossible to reproduce, were useful to the superpower on the brink of war with the Soviet Union. Justice for the victims of Unit 731 proved completely disposable. In granting the liberty of the men of Unit 731, and in collecting and using their data, the U.S. government morally inherited the cost in human lives and unspeakable suffering inexorably embedded within that horrific body of work. The State Department vigorously, albeit unsuccessfully, opposed the government's decision on the Unit 731 criminals, properly citing the abandonment of moral principle. The encyclopedic record of these experiments, the debate for punishing its authors and the immoral outcome of it, did not become widely known outside of Japan until the late 1980s.

Many of these scientists and physicians from Unit 731 went on to prominent and rewarding careers in Japanese biomedical industries, government agencies, and academia. Those men erected a shrine in Tokyo dedicated to the men of Unit 731 who died during the war. They also held festive annual reunions.

One former soldier assigned to Unit 731 in China, Yoshio Shinozuka, described in a 2002 BBC television documentary how he scrubbed the torsos of prisoners before the doctors sliced them open while they were conscious and without anesthesia. The treatment of the prisoners disturbed him at first, but he reported becoming accustomed to it. The old man Yoshio expressed deep remorse and was brought to tears by recollection of his actions as a fifteen-year-old soldier. Anita McNaught of the BBC also interviewed Unit 731 veteran Toshimi Mizobuchi, who admitted to killing many Chinese prisoners for experiments. She asked him, "Was there ever a time when you thought the work you were doing at Unit 731 was wrong, was inhumane?" His response: "No."

A landmark 1989 book by Peter Williams and David Wallace, *Unit 731: Japan's Secret Biological Warfare in World War II*, details the reach and depth of depravity of this grotesque history. According to those authors, a detachment of Unit 731 may have operated at Bandung in West Java, presumably at the former Pasteur Institute in that city— the site of the manufacture of the vaccine injections that killed the nine hundred romusha whose deaths were attributed to Mochtar. Although Ishii apparently visited that facility, there has been no evidence that biological weapons were developed there.

If Unit 731 indeed operated at the Pasteur Institute at Bandung, it would likely have been in the business of vaccines development and production—the core technical capacity of that facility prior to its seizure by the Japanese, and certainly a key biostrategic activity under the broader remit of Unit 731. The American government had no interest in the data on vaccines. Their own work in this arena was far more advanced. And it is very unlikely that any deal cut with Ishii would have involved activities in Indonesia. Further, the prosecution of war crimes committed in Indonesia fell almost entirely to the Dutch, British, and Australian military authorities. The Americans were not directly involved.

Finally, in the case of Mochtar and the murdered romusha, no serious legal challenge appears to have been mounted. No Japanese officer involved in these murders would have been put into a position where barter was necessary. Their crime simply went unexamined and unpunished. It seems likely that swamped Allied prosecutors would have chosen not to pursue indictments over the dead romusha at the Klender camp outside Jakarta on the weight of Mochtar's false confession (and his inability to retract it). Mochtar's murderers were among the many other sharks swimming through the Allied net of justice.

The telling of Mochtar's story aims at undoing this injustice and setting straight this record of Japan's era of Indonesian occupation. Exculpating Mochtar is important, but so is turning over the rock under which the real murderers have remained hidden in utter silence for seven decades, perhaps convinced that their crime no longer mattered or, even worse, that killing those romusha and Mochtar was no more than a patriotic defense of the Japanese homeland.

TWO

Politics and Science

The Truth

The truth is often raw, inconvenient, embarrassing, or dangerous. Science doesn't care about any of that. What people feel about revealed truth is irrelevant. The only matter of importance is its veracity. Once verified, that truth is immutable and nonnegotiable as reality. But the truth in politics is another matter. It often hinges on human feelings and perception of reality. The veracity of truth weighs relatively little. The raw truth can be cooked to taste. The histories of nations abound in examples of this culinary tradition.

In the 1980s Congress ordered scientific studies on the relationship between exposure to the herbicide Agent Orange and conditions of disease in veterans of the war in Vietnam exposed to the chemicals. Ill veterans prompted that investigative effort by going to their congressmen in substantial numbers with a variety of maladies they attributed to exposure to that chemical soup. Science obliged the congressmen and presented firm evidence demonstrating risk of cancers among those veterans as being indistinguishable from that in people never exposed to Agent Orange.[1] The veterans had real illnesses, but none could be scientifically linked to exposure to the chemicals. Congress nonetheless ordered compensation paid to exposed veterans suffering medical complaints.[2] What most Americans felt—that the government owed these ill veterans compensation for their service and sacrifices—overruled the verifiable facts negating the basis of their claim. The truth in politics is mutable

and negotiable, with political expediency or exigency often dispos-
ing with verified truth and its honest management.

This fact aids in grasping the Mochtar affair and its consequences,
including those touching us today. Japanese insistence upon a noble
war of self-defense against European imperialism and of the "divine"
nature of those who perished in doing so affects each of us directly
and profoundly. Mochtar's experience at the hands of those forces
reveals to us their true character and intent. His loss to such deceit
can and should instruct us to combat the cheating of truth from history, be it embarrassing, inconvenient, or dangerous.

Physician scientist Achmad Mochtar, among the brightest and
most valued citizens of occupied Netherlands East Indies, found himself cornered in a nexus of brutish wartime politics and the cause
of science. He became the scapegoat for a high-stakes political ploy
pitting the expediencies of ruthless men against an ugly truth they
owned. They accused Mochtar of a depraved crime: the deliberate
murder of hundreds of his fellow Indonesians as a way to shame
and politically undermine the occupiers of Indonesia. It was their
mass murder, but Mochtar could be blamed and presented as the
perpetrator. What people believed vastly outweighed the truth. This
book seeks that truth and deconstructs the lies conjured to conceal
its dangerous consequences.

Discovery of that truth, in the absence of much of the direct evidence that would support it, requires engaging and understanding the complexities of Indonesian history, politics, and the forty
months of Japanese occupation. The nature of the political relationship between the occupied and their occupier is key, and understanding it is necessary in grasping the swirl of currents we refer to
collectively as the Mochtar affair (a term we borrowed from Theodore Friend, a scholar of Indonesian history).

Further, we must delve into a very specific field of medicine, vaccination against tetanus, with fine-grained medical technical detail.
Vaccination was the instrument of the murder of the nine hundred
romusha at the camp at Klender outside Jakarta in early August
1944. Understanding why that vaccine was important to the Japanese and how it works will illuminate the motivation as well as the
modus operandi of the murderers. Further, these technical details

Politics and Science

reveal both the implausibility of manufacturing accident and the great likelihood of inhumane medical experimentation as the root cause of the deaths of the romusha at Klender.

A Dangerous and Delicate Liaison

Most Indonesians welcomed the eviction of the Dutch. The fact that the liberators neatly fit with Joyoboyo's prophecies about events that would lead to self-rule surely amplified the enthusiasm that met the arrival of the Imperial Japanese armed forces. Nowhere else in their new realm did the Japanese enjoy such a reception, and they did not fail to see the opportunities this presented them for managing occupied Indonesia with relative ease.

Only in Indonesia did the occupiers have a broad and attentive audience for their vision of "co-prosperity" for Asian peoples in the wake of the eviction of the Europeans and Americans. Further, few other of their holdings offered as great a supply of diverse strategic commodities for Japan and its armed forces. In Indonesia especially, the Japanese had conspicuous strategic interests at stake in sustaining the illusion of co-prosperity, that is to say, an occupation in the better interests of Indonesia and Indonesians.

At first glance, this does not seem to square with the copiously documented brutality of the Japanese occupation in Indonesia. The Indonesians welcomed the Japanese, politically and materially supporting their broader war aims against European and American colonial imperialism in the region. Why conduct a brutal occupation of a friendly nation? This apparent conflict derives in part from failing to see just what Indonesia was then and is now—a remarkably heterogeneous grouping of people. In 1942 the active Indonesian nationalists alone composed distinct democratic-, royalist-, Islamist-, and communist-leaning ideological factions. Other Indonesians remained loyal to the Dutch and were considered overt enemies by both the Japanese and the nationalists. Stern rule and violence against such enemies was both expected and largely tolerated by the nationalists. Most Indonesians saw the Japanese as an instrument in shaping whatever future Indonesia each faction had in mind. The lone exception was the communists. The Japanese had no tolerance for their ideology, so they melted quietly into the masses and avoided provoking the occupiers. Their rise and fall would come later, in 1965, Soekarno's "year of living dangerously."

The apparent conflict of a brutal occupation of a friendly nation also derives from the raw fact that the Japanese were not interested in seeing a free and independent Indonesia. They aimed squarely for colonial mastery of the East Indies following victory in the Pacific War. The occupation authorities leveraged the illusion of freedom and independence in maneuvering the incipient nation toward an enduring and complete subordination to Imperial Japan. Their wholesale enslavement and slaughter of Indonesians of almost every creed was part and parcel of achieving that vision. Only as defeat drew closer and finally inevitable, and with a vision of empire ruined by the vengeful Americans, did the Japanese in Indonesia speak earnestly of independence.

In early 1942 the Japanese occupation authorities courted those nationalists they found ideologically tolerable and useful. By Japanese lights, "useful" meant helpful in quelling and pacifying as much of the Indonesian populace as possible. The occupying forces created the idea of a four-leaf clover, with each nationalist faction represented by a leaf, all of them supported by the Japanese stem.

The Japanese pragmatically favored the leaf offering the greatest utility—the democratic faction led by the charismatic Javanese firebrand Soekarno, who was widely seen as the "Ratu Adil" (Just King) of the Joyoboyo prophesies. A gifted orator, Soekarno commanded the passions of most Indonesians. As an uncompromising and long-suffering nationalist, he deplored the Dutch, who had held him in prison. Soekarno often spoke publically of his gratitude to the Imperial Japanese for forcibly evicting the whites from the Asian sphere. Soekarno's political alignment to that end connected him and, by proxy, most Indonesians with Imperial Japan.

Soekarno tolerated the occupation and strived to keep himself in the good graces of its authors, but he would never have accepted this as the permanent condition the Japanese had in mind. His nationalist bona fides were genuine and concrete. They dominated his private view of the Japanese as a temporary necessity—a view hardened by Joyoboyo's prophecies. In the end, the Allied victory precluded what would certainly have been a cataclysmic falling out between

Soekarno and the Japanese occupiers. As events turned, the Japanese evicted the Dutch, Soekarno held his bile, and the Americans evicted the Japanese by forcing their surrender at Tokyo.

In the enormous wake of the Pacific War, Soekarno created the nation he long dreamed of, even at the cost of the long, bloody war between 1945 and 1949 when the Dutch returned to claim their colony. This success was not spontaneous, assured, or easily managed. Soekarno had to exercise extraordinary political skill in satisfying the occupied masses that the Japanese were not what they in fact were: a vastly harsher and more avaricious colonial exploiter than the Dutch. Much hinged on this deception, known by the Japanese to be an illusion, and hoped by Soekarno and most other Indonesians to be the temporary hardship described in *Pralembang Joyoboyo*. Given Soekarno's devout and massive following, both he and the Japanese understood that he could not simply be liquidated without enormous risk of rebellion and deep cost in goodwill. He was thus not entirely a puppet of the Japanese but a powerful force with which they had to reckon.

Nonetheless, Soekarno repeatedly expressed his sense of vulnerability during the occupation in his authorized 1965 biography, *Sukarno*, coauthored by Cindy Adams. Indeed, the Japanese did attempt to assassinate Mohammad Hatta (who became Soekarno's first vice president) in a clumsy arranged automobile accident in the mountains of West Java.[3] Hatta viewed the Japanese with far deeper skepticism and impatience than his compatriot, and he had expressed such views to too many people.

Soekarno and Hatta on the Mochtar Affair

Concern for the fate of Achmad Mochtar before and after his execution reached the highest echelons of indigenous political power in occupied Indonesia. He was firmly connected within that network of influence. Soekarno and Hatta, at the pinnacle of influence in that period, held diametrically opposed views on the arrest and execution of Mochtar. Each spoke on the record of the Mochtar affair long after the war, with Soekarno professing Mochtar's guilt of mass murder and Hatta suggesting that Mochtar had been unjustly accused and convicted.[4]

Hatta's instincts were correct. He knew Mochtar and understood how completely implausible it was that he might commit mass murder of any sort, much less against his fellow Indonesians. Further, Hatta more freely questioned and challenged the intentions of the occupier with respect to both Mochtar and the far broader context—and nearly paid for that stance with his life. For example, in a public speech in December 1942 Hatta expressed his joy at Indonesia being freed of the Dutch colonial yoke, but pointedly added that if another foreign power were to colonize the islands, he would rather see them all swallowed up by the sea. Hatta understood the Japanese as a malevolent and threatening presence and was aware of their deep stake in concealing that fact. Soekarno, on the other hand, was more deeply vested in concealment of Japanese wrongdoing. His alliance with the Japanese, they had ensured, was crystal clear to his following masses. He was shrewdly put into a position of political accountability for Japanese actions, including the romusha program in the broadest context and the event at Klender at the heart of the Mochtar affair. Thus the key to understanding Soekarno's assertion of Mochtar's guilt is the disputed crime itself, committed against nine hundred romusha.

The fact that those victims were romusha underpins the essential political dimension of the Mochtar affair. In collaboration with Indonesian political elites, the Japanese created a system of recruiting young Javanese men to "enlist" in the romusha corps for labor, mostly served among Indonesia's scattered islands. Enlisting was promoted much as it was in the United States or United Kingdom for joining the armed forces—implored and promoted by national leaders as patriotic duty. Soekarno was an avid promoter of the romusha program, reasoning that victory for Japan was victory for Indonesia (repulsing and defeating the white colonialists).[5] He was not likely to have fully known at the time what awaited the romusha at their work sites, and the failure of most to return home during the war could have been rationalized as the ongoing urgency of their labors.

What Soekarno and his associates could see of the program, largely at the railhead holding camps on Java, gave little indication of the cruel treatment awaiting these men at remote sites. The romusha at the transit camps on Java had been fed, provided medical care, and decently housed, albeit under armed guard ostensibly for their own protection against saboteurs. Such humane treatment was a deliberate ruse to protect the illusion of beneficence by the occupier and the popular support of nationalist leaders enabling the labor program. Upon arrival at their work sites—beyond the eyes of most important Indonesians—the romusha found that their living and working conditions deteriorated immediately and dramatically. Most of them would not survive. Soekarno expressed after the war some awareness of the harsh treatment of romusha at the time, but he viewed their suffering much as a national leader would of soldiers enlisted and lost in defense of the nation.

The truth of what happened would have destroyed the ruse of humane treatment and Japanese beneficence. As such, it was politically toxic to both the Japanese occupiers and to Soekarno, during the occupation and much later. His documented discussion with Cindy Adams on this matter occurred in 1963 or 1964, nearly two decades after the defeat and exit of menacing Japanese forces. His assertion of Mochtar's guilt even at this removed time seems to affirm his continuing political vulnerability from his sponsorship of the romusha program and his naiveté toward—or concealment of—the truth of Japanese intention and behavior toward Indonesians.

This book does not aim to sully the venerated reputation of Soekarno, but instead aims to restore the reputation of Mochtar. Although Soekarno's decisions in the narrow context of this affair may be seen as opportunistic and callous, such calculations are almost universally characteristic of high-stakes politics. Soekarno obviously played the Japanese to his ends as much as they played him. His success and their ultimate failure certainly matter, and it favorably colors the judgment of his broader actions. A brief examination of the product of Soekarno's labors of 1942 to 1945 is thus informative.

The Legacy of Soekarno and Hatta

Soekarno and Hatta successfully fathered a great nation. The clay from which the Republic of Indonesia was sculpted still bears their ideological fingerprints at almost every fold and feature. They molded a democratic and pluralistic secular republic that now lives up to that noble foundational vision. In 2014 Indonesia is the most stable and vibrant democracy in Southeast Asia. Despite being home to a devout Muslim majority, it is firmly deliberate in not being an Islamic nation. Indonesia is a hugely diverse and firmly secular republic. It has always acted vigorously against those seen as undermining its unifying secularism. The long separatist war at Aceh in northern Sumatra, for example, ceased only in 2006 when Jakarta reluctantly conceded formal recognition of the legal force of Islamic sharia'a law in that province (a lone exception to constitutional mandate against such).

Indonesian national identity embraces its vast ethnic and religious diversity. The national motto is "Bhineka Tunggal Ika," or Unity in Diversity. As will be explained later, in 1908 medical students at Batavia created the very idea of "Indonesia" by defining this unifying principle. Soekarno and Hatta would be the men to construct the republic using that ideological blueprint.

The dominant political parties in Indonesia today that represent this ideology, Gerindra ("Gerakan Indonesia Raya," Great Indonesia Movement) and the Partai Democratic Indonesia–Perjuangan (PDIP, Democratic Party of Indonesia–of Struggle), proudly carry the secular and pluralistic banner formulated in 1908 and enshrined in the 1945 constitution for the republic.[6] Indeed, the leader of PDIP in 2014 is Megawati Soekarnoputri, a former president of the republic and Soekarno's daughter. Her father's portrait appears in much of the PDIP publicity material. Those two parties, with their respective coalitions of most others, contested each other for the office of president in July 2014.

The legacy of Soekarno and Hatta is sometimes challenged in Indonesia today. The communists are gone, and the royalists are virtually irrelevant, but the Islamists remain a viable and legitimate political counter to the secular vision of Soekarno and Hatta. They see a different Indonesia: one governed more by Islamic teachings and law and less by liberal secular principles. Many Islamist-leaning political parties express a will to amend the constitution to accommodate that ideology.[7] Indonesians happy with the 1945 constitution, Muslim or otherwise, fear that a truly Islamic republic (in the model of Pakistan, for example) could exclude non-Muslims as less than full citizens, causing divides that challenge the cohesiveness of an enormously diverse nation. The extreme of such struggle between religious and secular political ideologies among Muslims may be seen in the violent divisions tearing at Egypt in 2013.

Relatively few people live in the eastern half of the Indonesian archipelago, and most of them are Christian or animist. The famous tourism destination of Bali, which is the ancestral home of Soekarno's mother, is Hindu. Large Christian enclaves exist in Sumatra, Kalimantan, and Sulawesi. Christians, Buddhists, Hindus, and Confucianists live in substantial numbers all across overwhelmingly Muslim Java, as do pockets of ancient animist beliefs. Even within the Muslim fold, Ahmadi and Shi'ite sect minorities are scattered across Sunni-dominated islands.

What would a Sunni Islamic republic hold for Indonesia's many non-Muslims who inhabit much of the united archipelago? This key question dominated the thinking of Soekarno and especially Hatta and their largely Muslim compatriots in forging the secular Republic of Indonesia—a nation not divided by culture, language, or religion, but united in their inherent broad diversity and identity as being uniquely Indonesian. The one concession they made to bring the Islamists to this vision is the constitutional requirement that the president be Muslim. Islamist efforts to have the constitution recognize and validate Islamic laws, sharia'a according to Sunnis, as the law of the republic were successfully outflanked by Soekarno and Hatta and their allies. At a critical moment in May 1945, Hatta shrewdly pointed to Ataturk's secularism in Muslim Turkey as the best model for a modern nation. Hatta may be rightfully credited as the driving intellectual force of national unity by secularism for Indonesia.

This struggle of national identity is not entirely decided, and conflicts still arise, both serious and silly. A hardline Indonesian Islamist minority publicly threatened the Miss World beauty pageant held in Bali in 2013. They considered such a public display of feminine beauty an unacceptable affront to Islam, despite the concession by organizers to dispense with the traditional bikini segment of the competition. The Islamists vowed to disrupt the competition and gathered at the port on Java that offers ferry service to nearby Bali—a line of female police officers (backed by large cadres of male officers standing by) denied them access to the ferry. The Hindu Balinese marveled at such an audacious infringement upon their perception of what is moral or an affront to their own distinct culture and religion. Various Balinese officials, including its governor, vowed the show would go on, and it did. This rather absurd conflict illustrates how the secular ideological glue applied by Soekarno and Hatta holds this diverse archipelago together as a unified nation.

Indonesia and Indonesians shall continue to decide their own political destiny. They have struggled hard and won their rights as citizens to vote their preferences. By all accounts their elections have uniformly been free and fair since the fall of Soekarno's successor, Soeharto, in 1998. Although on a number of fronts Soekarno (and Soeharto) did not live up to the legacy of the constitution that the republic's first president and vice president enshrined, it exists today thanks to them. That constitution should be viewed not as embodying any man and his human flaws but as the blended vision of Soekarno and his compatriots for the future of a diverse nation which embraces and protects all citizens rather than solely a dominant majority—the watermark of greatness among modern societies. The chronic racial and religious conflicts that punctuate modern Malaysian politics and governance may be viewed as a stark contrast to the Indonesian model.

The favorable fate of the Republic of Indonesia, set in the template delivered by Soekarno and his allies, does not excuse Soekarno's treatment of Mochtar, but perhaps aids in understanding it. Abu Hanifah (nephew of Mochtar, Dutch Navy medical officer, revolutionary commando, minister, and ambassador) in his *Tales of a Revolution*, penned in the early 1970s, presents a very harsh view of Soekarno and his management of the romusha and of the Mochtar affair. The Republic of Indonesia of the 1960s and 1970s is very different from the same nation forty years later in most important social, economic, and political dimensions. It is more fair, prosperous, and open than ever in its history. So some degree of forgiveness of Soekarno may rightfully emerge from a genuine and well-deserved national gratitude. In the final analysis, Soekarno did not kill the romusha or Mochtar—a ruthless occupier did. Acknowledging these wrongs does not diminish the realized vision of Soekarno and Hatta's Indonesia Raya.

What Happened at Klender?

Nine hundred romusha died from acute tetanus poisoning in early August 1944 at a railhead encampment at Klender just outside Jakarta. Within several days of receiving en masse vaccination—allegedly against dysentery, typhus, and cholera—all the romusha were gripped by the rigor and grimace of acute tetanus. All were dead within seventy-two hours of the first onset of symptoms.

After two months of investigation and contemplation, the Japanese asserted that Mochtar, as the director of the Eijkman Institute in Jakarta, along with the scientists working under his direction, had deliberately placed tetanus toxin in the vaccine administered to the romusha. They had done so, according to the Kenpeitai, to discredit the Japanese and undermine their war effort.

All were arrested in early October 1944, along with the three doctors from the municipal health service who administered the vaccinations. They were held at the Kenpeitai jail in central Jakarta. Almost all were brutally and repeatedly tortured. One doctor died under particularly savage torture, and his mutilated remains were paraded before the prisoners. In early December 1944, in a rare moment when speaking was possible, Mochtar told at least three fellow captives that their release was imminent but that he would not be freed and probably would not survive.

All of the Eijkman scientists except Mochtar were released by January 1945 and not further molested. The two surviving municipal health service doctors were transferred to regular prisons. Dr. Mohammad Ali Hanafiah, Mochtar's brother-in-law, would later pen a powerful memoir of his experience, certainly the key body of evidence for understanding the depth of horror of the Mochtar affair. Dr. Marzoeki also committed to paper his experience at the hands of the Kenpeitai—and a memoir by his daughter, Latifah Kodijat-Marzoeki, corroborates Hanafiah's testimony.

Mochtar agreed to sign a confession affirming the Japanese account of the event at Klender. Evidence suggests he did so in order to save his colleagues, bartering their release for his signature. That signature sealed his appointment with a sword at that ugly tree on the waterfront. His murder, as Mochtar certainly understood, would silence the looming and inevitable postwar Allied query on the deadly event at Klender.

The Indonesian medical community remembers Mochtar as a martyr. A major public hospital at Bukit Tinggi, Sumatra, not far from his place of birth, bears his name. Since the fall of Soekarno in late 1965, none give credence to the confession or the Japanese accounting of events painting him as a mass murderer. Indeed, in the 1970s President Soeharto recognized Mochtar's martyrdom with an honorary award. However, what exactly happened at Klender has until now eluded clarity. Many Indonesians (and foreign historians) familiar with the available details suppose that there was an accidental adulteration of the dysentery/typhus/cholera vaccine with tetanus during manufacture by the Japanese army at the former Pasteur Institute at Bandung. They view the Japanese actions against Mochtar as an attempt to avoid the embarrassment of having their medical men perceived as incompetent.

This book examines that hypothesis of an accident of manufacture and rejects it. If Mochtar did not sabotage the vaccine administered at Klender, and if accidental contamination during production does not explain what happened, what does? How could the vaccine have contained tetanus, either the bacterium or its toxin, both of which were capable of the same fatal result?

In answering that question we first need to understand tetanus and its treatment or prevention by vaccination. We will also examine the importance of the vaccine to Japanese soldiers, its very short supply, and the improbability of the Japanese administering such a precious medication to disposable romusha. We shall also carefully examine a separate, thoroughly documented incident involving the accidental killing of fifteen condemned Indonesian prisoners in trying to demonstrate the efficacy of a tetanus vaccine improvised by the Japanese navy at Surabaya in East Java in January 1945.

These lines of evidence frame a different hypothesis for what happened at Klender. The Japanese army vaccine makers at Bandung, like their navy counterparts in Surabaya, improvised a tetanus vaccine and, with Allied invasion and heavy combat fully anticipated at any time, they acted to develop immediate evidence that the vaccine actually worked.

We believe that the Japanese army doctors at the former Pasteur Institute at Bandung first vaccinated the romusha at Klender and then challenged them with tetanus toxin, probably with misplaced confidence that their improvised vaccine would protect these human guinea pigs. The ugly shock of their deaths rippled widely and with deep political ramifications for the occupiers.

In Mochtar, the Kenpeitai found a viable solution to this very serious political problem. The fashioned him into a saboteur and executed him to protect that lie and, later, their personal liberty.

The Empire Strikes

The beginning to Mochtar's tragic end was the Imperial Japanese attack at Pearl Harbor on December 7, 1941. This attack, albeit directly on the United States, did not form part of a strategy for conquering the United States. It was instead aimed at crippling the only military asset that could upset Japan's planned conquest of Southeast Asia and Australia. To win that objective Japan needed unchallenged command of the seas of all of East Asia. The asset most capable of posing a challenge to their plans happened to be the American Pacific Fleet moored at Pearl Harbor. Success in eliminating that threat was prerequisite to the absolute domination over the entire Asian sphere that Imperial Japan craved.

Japan's belligerence in Asia predated Pearl Harbor. Their seizure of Korea occurred in 1910, and the intrusions upon China began in 1931 with the occupation of Manchuria. The frank invasion of China commenced in 1937. However, until Pearl Harbor, Japan did not seriously threaten Southeast Asia, even though they managed to seize Vietnam from the French in late 1940 through Vichy France–Nazi Germany–Imperial Japan alliances.

The next chapter of this book details the collapse of colonial Southeast Asia beginning on December 7, 1941, and the inhumane means of Japanese assertion of dominion over those conquests. A military understanding of those events reveals the arrant absurdity and perfidy of the claim that European imperialistic aggression against the Japanese homeland caused the Pacific War. The bungling management of the military forces of the colonial powers in Asia, much less their neglected and inadequate state, cannot be reconciled to an offensive military posture at the time. Those forces had been defensively positioned long before the Japanese offensive that completely annihilated them. The Europeans and Americans in Asia, or their Chinese allies, did not plot invasion or subjugation of Japan until after the vast Japanese military offensive. The "heroic self-defense of the Japanese motherland" was, in fact, an amoral force-of-arms conquest by a militaristic fascist power bent upon subjugating Asia in the cause of advancing the Japanese race at deep costs to all others. Those actions alone caused the Allies to recover, rally, and crush the Imperial Japanese. The reverence and respect at Yasukuni shown for the men who plotted and carried out the vast array of crimes against humanity in their Pacific War affronts the truth of responsibility and the millions of victims. Silent tolerance of or acquiescence to such a deceit and injustice deeply erodes our humanity.

THREE

Beginning of the End

Midnight for Netherlands East Indies: December 1941 to April 1942

In the early 1600s the Dutch East India Company, the voc, wrested economic and military control of key pieces of the Indonesian archipelago from the Portuguese (excepting East Timor) and various indigenous kingdoms and sultanates. Before the century ended, they successfully, and rather brutally, contested the British for possession of the fabled Spice Islands of Maluku.[1] Total domination eluded the Dutch in some enclaves. Bali, for example, resisted Dutch control until a military invasion and subjugation in the early 1900s.[2] But Dutch mastery in playing local rivalries to advantage paved the way to a colonial domination of the Indonesian archipelago that lasted over three centuries.

The colonial military citadel in Southeast Asia that protected the Netherlands East Indies in 1941–shared by British and American armed forces at Malaya, Borneo, and the Philippines—completely collapsed in the 114 days between December 7, 1941, and April 1, 1942. If you can imagine a 322-year Dutch dominance of the archipelago as a single 24-hour day, those four months may be considered the final minute in that colonial day. In this minute, events corresponding to twelve bell tolls at midnight heralded the end of that colonial day.

In December 1941 Abu Hanifah, nephew of Achmad Mochtar and a chronicler of this period in Indonesia's history, was serving as a commissioned medical officer in the Dutch navy aboard the *Plancius*. He described the call his ship made at Singapore harbor on December 7, just hours before the Japanese attacked Pearl Harbor, "For the first time in my life I saw two huge battleships. They were the *Prince of Wales* and the *Repulse*. These two ships were just steaming out and passed us at a distance of a hundred feet. The Dutch on board our ship were jubilant: 'Look at those ships,' they said, 'the Japanese will think twice before they attack us.' Indeed the ships looked so formidable, so unconquerable."[3] The extreme vulnerability of such warships to air power, unknown up to that day in history, would very soon be decisively demonstrated.

The first bell toll of colonial midnight in Southeast Asia sounded with the unprovoked surprise attack by carrier-borne Japanese warplanes early in the morning of Sunday, December 7, 1941, against the idle American Pacific Fleet at Pearl Harbor in distant Hawaii.

News of the Japanese success at Pearl Harbor streaked through Imperial Japan's military commands coded as "Tora. Tora. Tora." Those words launched planned air raids on American air bases on Luzon in the Philippines. The conquest of Southeast Asia was under way.

Formosa-based Japanese warplanes carried out those attacks just eight hours after Pearl Harbor. Heavy fog had delayed their launch by six hours. Nonetheless, by midday on December 8, most American air assets on Luzon had been destroyed. Now facing no real threat from the air, a waiting seaborne invasion force landed at Luzon the same day, sounding the second bell toll of colonial midnight.

Early in the morning of December 10, the third bell sounded: the *Prince of Wales* and *Repulse*, along with their destroyer escorts, were sunk in a matter of minutes by waves of Japanese torpedo- and dive-bombers. The British had not yet absorbed the lesson so painfully inflicted upon the American navy at Pearl Harbor: the tactical threat of air power against surface warships of any tonnage or firepower.

The British flotilla had steamed haughtily out of Singapore with friendly air cover that was both scant and obsolete. Superior Japanese warplanes and tactics quickly brushed those defenses aside and destroyed the British flotilla with ease. Japanese amphibious forces then landed on the Malay Peninsula virtually unopposed.

The Allies all across the region had arrogantly and fatally underestimated Japanese military equipment, skill, audacity, and ferocity.

It was to prove a catastrophic failure of responsibility to those most reliant upon them—the peoples they had colonized.

Through December and January, Gen. Tomoyuki Yamashita's 30,000 front-line troops raced down the Malay Peninsula toward Singapore, sounding the fourth bell toll. They poured through poorly organized and outfitted British and Australian defenders—most of whom hastily retreated to Singapore. At the last moment, the British blasted the causeway that connected the mainland peninsula to the island of Singapore at its tip. Yamashita—now called the "Tiger of Malaya"—paused for a long precious week to collect his troops and supplies, unmolested by the reeling Allies. A forlorn fifth bell toll then sounded.

Singapore could only brace and wait. The big guns defending her were outfitted uselessly, their ordnance suited only for attacking heavy warships. Contrary to popular myth, it was possible for the big guns at Singapore to fire toward Yamashita's positions on the peninsula. However, the only type of shells they had would simply burrow into the ground before exploding harmlessly. The big guns may as well have been pointed at the empty sea. No Allied military capacity or asset could harass the Japanese forces resting, resupplying, and glowering at Singapore across the narrow straits.

Lt. Gen. Arthur Percival, commanding the amassed Allied forces at Singapore, had been ordered to make a stand and to absolutely reject the idea of a general surrender. Prime Minister Winston Churchill cabled to Percival's commander, Gen. Archibald Wavell, just after Yamashita had crossed the straits on February 8, 1942:

> I think you ought to realise the way we view the situation in Singapore. It was reported to Cabinet by the C.I.G.S. [Chief of the Imperial General Staff, Gen. Alan Brooke] that Percival has over 100,000 [sic] men, of whom 33,000 are British and 17,000 Australian. It is doubtful whether the Japanese have as many in the whole Malay Peninsula. . . . In these circumstances the defenders must greatly outnumber Japanese forces who have crossed the straits, and in a well-contested battle they should destroy them. There must at this stage be no thought of saving the troops or sparing the population. The battle must be fought to the bitter end at all costs. The 18th Division has a chance

to make its name in history. Commanders and senior officers should die with their troops. The honour of the British Empire and of the British Army is at stake. I rely on you to show no mercy to weakness in any form. With the Russians fighting as they are and the Americans so stubborn at Luzon, the whole reputation of our country and our race is involved. It is expected that every unit will be brought into close contact with the enemy and fight it out.[4]

Churchill's gift with language conveys the gravity with which the sole remaining Allied European power viewed the rapidly unfolding and deteriorating events in East Asia. Yet London is very far from Singapore, and despite the prime minister's urgency and lofty call to martyrdom, the situation had become desperate. Japanese infiltrators had guided their attacks to strategically critical sites like Bukit Timah, where most ammunition and fuel had been stored and where the supply of water to the city could be cut off. On February 15, 1942, despite direct orders from Wavell not to do so, Percival signed an unconditional general surrender to Yamashita. The sixth bell toll sounded.

An enraged Churchill in London never forgave Percival this humiliation of the British armed forces: surrendering nearly 100,000 entrenched defenders to a logistically stretched invader of 30,000 troops. When the war was drawing to a close in mid-1945, the recently liberated General Percival was flown to the Philippines to sit at the proverbial turned table, where he witnessed Yamashita's unconditional surrender to Douglas MacArthur. After the signing, Percival refused to shake the conquered general's hand, causing Yamashita to break down in tears.

The carnage inflicted upon the civilian populace of Manila by Yamashita's troops in early 1945 as the Americans closed in formed the basis of the war tribunal charges against him. Yamashita was condemned to hang. He penned a plea to MacArthur to be shot like a soldier rather than hung as a criminal. That request was denied with the assertion that he was indeed a criminal and not a soldier.

In the besieged Philippines in early 1942, the Americans spared Manila by declaring it an open city. They had retreated to their strongholds on the Bataan Peninsula and Corregidor Island in Manila Bay.

Yamashita's orders to his troops to do precisely the same maneuver in 1945 had been ignored by elements of his command. Those Japanese conducted wholesale slaughter and rape of tens of thousands of civilian Filipinos until the Americans finally cornered and killed most of them in their Spanish fortress redoubt at Intramuros in the center of old Manila.

American jurists credibly questioned the legality of Yamashita's conviction. Appeal of it went to the United States Supreme Court and was upheld, but the two dissenting justices (of seven deciding) described his looming execution as a "lynching." In that light some may view Yamashita as one of the few Japanese military men perhaps meriting the homage paid him as a martyr at Yasukuni. However, few survivors of the fall of Singapore, as one example, would ascribe to this notion—troops under Yamashita's direct command slaughtered between five and ninety thousand unarmed Chinese Singaporean civilians in the Sook Ching massacres in the days following Percival's surrender. Those massacres also occurred at uncountable rural villages all along the Malay Peninsula, where ethnic Chinese families were separated from their Malay neighbors and taken into the forest and murdered by sword and bayonet—hundreds of families slain together. *Sook Ching* roughly translates as "ethnic cleansing." On the day before Percival's surrender, February 14, Japanese troops slaughtered 320 defenseless patients and clinical staff (men, women, and children, European and Singaporean alike) by bayonet and sword at the Alexandra Hospital in Singapore. In one surgical suite the Japanese soldiers barged in and slew the patient on the operating table, then turned their swords upon the protesting surgical team. Such was the heroic defense of the Japanese motherland. Yamashita was not tried for these and other horrific crimes. In the case of the slaughter at the Alexandra Hospital, Yamashita did immediately arrest and execute the Japanese officers who carried it out.

Though the Americans at Bataan and Corregidor in early 1942 would fight desperately through April, no relief was possible and surrender to the Japanese on Luzon was inevitable. The Philippines had been effectively lost by the failure to repulse the invasion in early December and by the retreat of the American Asiatic Fleet from Philippine waters, which left Japanese resupply and reinforcements unchallenged.

With Singapore captured and secure by mid-February 1942, Japanese troops promptly launched invasions at Sumatra (Bangka and Palembang), Borneo (Tarakan), and the Celebes (Manado) during the last two weeks of that month. Netherlands East Indies began to crumble, the seventh bell toll of colonial midnight.

On February 27 and 28 remnants of the American, British, Australian, and Dutch naval fleets in Asia gathered at Batavia and Surabaya on the north coast of Java for a last stand. In the historically obscure but strategically critical Battle of the Java Sea, numerically superior and more modern Japanese warships decisively crushed the substantial Allied flotilla, with few ships escaping. The modern Dutch light cruiser *De Ruyter* went down with Admiral of the Fleet van Doorn. The American heavy cruiser *Houston* (christened at launch by Franklin D. Roosevelt) and the British cruiser *Exeter*, both crippled and trying to escape to Australia through the Sunda Strait between Java and Sumatra, were each attacked and sunk on its approach. The Asiatic naval fleets of the colonial powers—neglected and inadequate—had been annihilated. The eighth bell of colonial midnight rang.

The Dutch on Java received this news with shock and disbelief. Now the entire East Indies lay naked against the Imperial Japanese juggernaut. They had only hours to contemplate this turn of events—the Japanese war machine arrived the very next day to claim its lush prize and all of her strategically valuable materials. On the first day of March, the Empire of Japan's Sixteenth Army landed forces on the island of Java (at Banten and Indramayu), the political and economic heart of the vast East Indies archipelago. The ninth bell sounded.

In just one week, that force of roughly 35,000 troops, most of them on bicycles or in commandeered sedans, swept through Batavia and on to Bandung in the volcanic mountains of West Java, where they won the surrender of 93,000 Dutch Indies troops on March 9: the tenth bell toll.

The eleventh and the twelfth rang with the capture of Maluku and then Dutch New Guinea a few short weeks later. Dutch colonial possession of these astonishingly rich tropical islands thus ignominiously ended. Imperial Japan now commanded Indonesia's wealth of oil, rubber, nickel, iron, copper, coal, timber, quinine, rice, and people.

Banzai

The Japanese military clique was deeply surprised by the ease with which such extraordinary wealth could be seized. The Dutchmen, with whom they earlier had unsuccessfully tried to negotiate for trade in strategic commodities, were now either dead, fleeing, or in prison camps. A new day had dawned, one dominated by the battle flag of the Rising Sun. In April 1942 "Banzai!" (a victory cry meaning "ten thousand years") rang out across the vast new southern fringe of the empire.

Lt. Gen. Imamura Hitoshi commanded the Sixteenth Army. His troops were veterans toughened by five years of warfare in China. The emperor's finest had been dispatched to capture this jewel called the East Indies. Many of them would be quickly moved eastward to Guadalcanal in the Solomon Islands to check the American counterattack on their sweeping advance that threatened to encircle and ultimately invade Australia. They would all be lost in that first confrontation with balanced American military might.

Though militarily conquered, the East Indies was a high-maintenance prize. There were nearly 200,000 Dutch civilians, the Dutch Indies army of 130,000, scattered thousands of the remnants of British, American, and Australian armed forces, and roughly 70 million indigenous people with no special affection for the emperor of Japan. There were obvious enemies to capture and imprison, an elite few on their list for execution, and an already entrenched Allied espionage network that had enlisted those locals who remained loyal to European masters. The Netherlands East Indies was far easier to seize than it was to manage and keep.

The Kenpeitai

General Imamura had a special tool attached to his Sixteenth Army to cope with those hostile currents. It was a very small fraction of his manpower on Java, just 30 officers and 492 warrant and noncommissioned officers, but it was a sharp and efficient tool nonetheless. This was the Third Field Kenpeitai Command fresh from

China, soon to be redesignated the Sixteenth Army Kenpeitai, under the command of Col. Kuzumi Kenzaburo.

They called themselves military police, but their usage of that term was not meant in the sense of being peace officers. They did not direct traffic, guard compounds, or arrest petty criminals. Apart from their black boots, black collar devices, and a white armband, they looked like any other Japanese soldier in uniform. The armband expressed three kanji characters, *ken pei tai*, that translate roughly as "military law officer." This elite cadre—feared even by high-ranking regular army officers—policed devotion to the emperor and the military clique surrounding him.

The Kenpeitai men, *kenpei*, closing in on their new base at Batavia (about to be renamed Jakarta), possessed the cruelest and most vicious loyalty to that clique in Tokyo. Their skill in cold-blooded murder was already well honed. They had played a direct hand in the national rise of the military as a dominant political entity. They had already imprisoned, tortured, and murdered thousands of fellow Japanese citizens who were—or simply seemed to be—hostile to their aims. Visiting death upon people they viewed as inferior races, especially those natives who dared oppose or threaten the empire, represented not even the slightest moral challenge. It was rather a duty they gladly undertook. Willingness to kill unflinchingly was a source of pride among kenpei ranks.

Beheading by sword, with its highly symbolic yet absolutely unambiguous demonstration of the fullest subordination possible, held a special significance. The Kenpeitai considered shooting or bayoneting as a means of murder brutish and below their dignity. Their organizational culture embraced the spirit of summary execution by sword. They invented a word for the practice: *kikosako.*

Arresting kenpei would invoke kikosako when faced with clear evidence of guilt or when the burden of judicial process seemed unsustainable or simply inconvenient. By their own recollections:

> Kenpeitai Headquarters [at Jakarta] became so overwhelmed by time constraints, the frequency of incidents, and a shortage of hands that we ended up being unable to afford the time to conduct court-martial proceedings scrupulously. Major Murase Mitsuo, chief of the Tokko

[literally, Thought Police] Division at the time, therefore received approval from Lieutenant General Harada Kumakichi to sentence or take severe measures with those whose investigations had been concluded and for whom suspicion had been established, without holding martial law proceedings. "Severe measures" meant execution, or "kikosako" as we Kenpeitai called it.[5]

Theodore Friend worked a translation of kikosako as "hell craft." The Kenpeitai fully understood and committed to their evil. Summary execution of defenseless prisoners by sword and many other means was encouraged, condoned, and institutionalized by the forces that invaded Java.

Although this history focuses upon the Jakarta Kenpeitai, the brutality of the Japanese occupation reached across the entire archipelago, throughout all of the forty months of occupation. An Indonesian friend and colleague of the authors reluctantly related a story of the occupation as a means of explaining his stern refusal to greet visiting Japanese scientists at Jakarta in the late 1980s. In 1942 he was a boy living near Pontianak, western Borneo, when the Japanese armed forces appeared. They forced all residents to the large town square, including women and children. All of the authorities of the town, Dutch and Indonesian alike, were then beheaded in the square, one by one. Japanese soldiers wielding poles watched the crowd, striking anyone who looked away. All were forced to witness exactly who was now unequivocally in charge of their affairs.

Abu Hanifah, in his memoir *Tales of a Revolution,* recounts the arrest of a Dr. Roebini at Pontianak. The Japanese considered him a threat, as they did many intellectuals, and had marked him for execution. His family had recently departed for Java to visit relatives, so the Japanese postponed the execution and summoned Mrs. Roebini and her two children back to Pontianak. They explained that Dr. Roebini was seriously ill and needed assistance. The Japanese then patiently awaited the return of Dr. Roebini's family. According to Hanifah, "Dr. Roebini and his wife were beheaded in front of their children. I saw these children afterwards and they were still in a kind of shock."[6]

This sort of brutality escapes comprehension, but knowing the capacity of the occupier for such inhumanity helps explain the sub-jugated behavior of the occupied. What would an Indonesian, forced to witness children seeing the heads of their parents sliced away, think of his chances of defiance against this sort of master? Such an effect would provide the obvious strategic intent of the Japanese: strict obedience by terror. Their sadism had purpose and function.

No one will ever know how many people fell victim to kikosako in Batavia, much less the East Indies as a whole or in the broader Pacific War. In late 1937, during the siege of Nanking in China, two Japanese sublieutenants, Mukai Toshiaki and Noda Takeshi, raced to see who could behead 100 people first. The *Japan Advertiser* ran this headline at the time, "Contest to Kill First 100 Chinese with Sword Extended When Both Fighters Exceed Mark—Mukai Scores 106 and Noda 105."[7] Japanese newspapers detailed their ensuing competition to outdo the other, much like coverage afforded competing athletic teams. Both men survived the war to be tried and executed by Chinese firing squads for these crimes. They, too, are honored at Yasukuni despite having been labeled war criminals.

The capacity of the Japanese armed forces that invaded the East Indies for such inhumanity had been cultivated in their invasion of China. These were the same men who invaded the East Indies. Iris Chang left us with a compelling account of that capacity in her book *The Rape of Nanking*, a body of work that alerted many in the West to the depth of depravity of the Imperial Japanese armed forces.[8] A diary entry of Japanese army doctor Hosaka Akira, assigned to an infantry unit (Third Infantry Battalion, Twentieth Regiment, Sixteenth Division in the Shanghai Expedition Army) closing in on Nanking, gives us some idea of that inhumanity:

> At 10:00 on 29 November 1937 we left to clean out the enemy in Chang Chou and at noon we entered the town. An order was received to kill the residents and eighty (80) of them, men and women of all ages, were shot to death [at dusk]. I hope this will be the last time I'll ever witness such a scene. The people were all gathered in one place. They were all praying, crying, and begging for help. I just couldn't bear watching such a pitiful spectacle. Soon the heavy machine guns opened fire and the sight of those people screaming and falling to the

ground is one I could not face even if I had had the heart of a monster. War is truly terrible.[9]

That Japanese medical officer delivered his diary to Allied War Tribunal prosecutors in the hope of justice for those victims. He did
not have the heart of a monster, but his commanders did.

Kenpei posted in Jakarta recalled after the war that Eurasians and
Chinese were particularly targeted with kikosako.[10] The Kenpeitai
viewed these two groups, with some accuracy, as especially loyal to
the Dutch. The Eurasians, especially those born to Dutch fathers,
were typically fiercely loyal to Holland. As for the Chinese, they had
thrived economically under Dutch administration of colonial affairs.
Further, they had obvious loyalties to China, their ancestral or actual
homeland, which was still stubbornly resisting military subjugation.

By July 1943, as the tide of war began to turn against them, the
Japanese became increasingly anxious about an Allied landing on
Java launched from Australia. Moreover, in that same month the
prime minister of Japan, Gen. Tojo Hideki, visited Jakarta and met
with Soekarno and his colleagues, promising them Indonesian participation in governance and greater freedoms.

The Kenpeitai viewed such promises as provocative of further disobedience. They saw value in launching a kikosako operation and
obtained the consent of the military command to do so. Over the
next couple of months, some 293 people, most of them Eurasian,
were summarily executed largely on the basis of hollow remarks by
Tojo. This was quickly followed, during November and December
1943, with another kikosako operation by the Kenpeitai across all of
Java and Sumatra, aimed at eliminating espionage networks. The
operation netted 1,468 people on Java and over 3,000 on Sumatra,
again most of them Eurasians.[11] It is not known how many of these
were actually executed, but Post estimates that in Sumatra alone at
least 350 were put to the sword.

Kenpeitai murder was certainly not limited to kikosako. They also
murdered according to their somewhat less freehanded martial law
proceedings. The headquarters of the Sixteenth Army was located
at Tanjung Priok, the port for Jakarta. This facility included their
"judicial" process infrastructure and a detachment of the Jakarta

Kenpeitai commanded by Maj. Taniguchi Kiyoshi. The Japanese established an execution ground nearby at Ancol to carry out death sentences meted out by martial law. That ground is preserved today as an honorary cemetery managed by a Dutch-Indonesian foundation, though most of those executed at Ancol were Indonesians. The cemetery sits directly on the Java Sea where Ancol adjoins Tanjung Priok.

So-called judicial executions occurred on this site from 1942 to 1945. According to the Dutch managers, the executions were conducted at a tree that today stands preserved just thirty meters from a monument to the victims. The site of that monument is where in September 1945 the Allies found a mass grave for the execution ground. The bodies of the executed had been dragged to a pit, then thrown in and covered in dirt. By war's end the pit had grown to become a conspicuous mound.

During the brief restoration of the Dutch government at Batavia, from September 1945 to December 1949, authorities excavated the mass grave at Ancol and tried, as best they could, to identify individual victims and to give each a decent burial away from the mass grave. They unearthed the remains of five hundred people, most unidentifiable. They obtained from the Japanese a list of the names of some of the executed. Those names now appear on placards around the cemetery. One of those placards reads "Prof. Dr. A. Mochtar."

End Game, Jakarta 1945

The last Kenpeitai execution at Ancol is lost to history. As any student of the Pacific War will attest, Imperial Japanese forces held the spirit of defeat at bay until the bitter end. On May 24, 1945, the Sixteenth Army on Java received these orders from the Seventh District Division of the Imperial Japanese Army Command: "Upon the enemy offensive, you must gradually weaken enemy strength everywhere and use your utmost force to crush their plan. Every effort must be made to secure the strategic areas of western Java as the circumstances compel it."[12]

Defeat was by then certain. U.S. forces were taking Okinawa in southern Japan, American heavy bombers attacked all major Japanese cities at will and without challenge, and the U.S. Navy had complete command of all sea lanes in the Pacific. Nevertheless, the military commanders of the empire of Japan aimed to inflict as much injury as physically possible. This may have been a strategic means of improving the position of Japan at a negotiation of surrender. However, the Allies had by this time made it clear to the government of Japan, through various channels, that nothing less than unconditional surrender would be accepted.

The morality of both positions may be questioned, but the futile tenacity of the Imperial Japanese may in large measure be blamed upon their bushido creed. Long before any thought of suing for peace entered the strategic equation, they had demonstrated a willingness to die rather than surrender. It is likely that the executions at Tanjung Priok, and elsewhere across the crumbled and ruined empire of Japan, continued up to and even after the official instrument of surrender was signed aboard the USS *Missouri* in Tokyo Bay on September 2, 1945.

The Japanese in Indonesia, from the first day of invasion, projected themselves as "big brother"—older, wiser, and taking charge out of a filial sense of devotion to a little brother who had been bullied by European exploiters. An instruction on Indonesian politics circulated as a top-secret document to Japanese army commanders in Indonesia in late 1944, as they dangled the independence carrot dangerously close to the mouth of the eager mule, reveals their sentiments: "We must instruct and guide them sternly like parents or older brothers or sisters."[13] The Japanese nonetheless commanded absolute authority in Indonesia, taking direct charge of almost every enterprise of importance. It was necessary to demonstrate to the Indonesian people at all levels a supremacy bordering on perfection. In Japanese eyes, and indeed many Indonesian eyes, the immediate and complete collapse of the Dutch in the East Indies had revealed the Europeans as incompetent frauds incapable of managing the affairs and welfare of the indigenous people of the East Indies. Right up to the moment of their unconditional surrender, Japanese strategies and tactics pivoted on what they felt was a social, political, and even military necessity to demonstrate infallibility to the Indonesian people.

The narrative history of this book illustrates a single yet profound and movingly human example of the effects of this tragically flawed reasoning. The Indonesian people were genuinely inferior to the

Imperial Japanese in only one important respect: they had fewer weapons and lacked enthusiasm for using them to terrorize and enslave others. Nor did they suffer the pathological racial vanity of the Imperial Japanese. Indonesians represented many races and hundreds of ethnic identities, and they had mixed with the Dutch over the centuries. For almost all of them, indifference to racial identity was an engrained second nature. But for the Imperial Japanese, like that of their Aryan allies in Germany, their racial identity and its supremacy above all others formed the very basis of their imperial ambitions. Challenge or compromise of their racial supremacy represented to them a very serious matter. Crushing any threat to this perception was fundamental to their war strategy and post-victory vision of empire.

The Kenpeitai were charged with ensuring that occupied peoples had correct thoughts about their Imperial Japanese masters. They dedicated a division specifically to this task—the Tokko. The Tokko would deal with any events that could potentially cause Indonesians to exhibit anything other than complete obedience to Japanese authority. Establishing the perception that they were perfect masters constituted a key ingredient in their management of thought and feeling. The Tokko took very seriously any incident that could incite Indonesians to see the Japanese as either flawed or perhaps not having their best interests in mind.

As the Mochtar affair began to unfold in Jakarta in early August 1944, the Kenpeitai stepped in aggressively to manage it. Their brutal actions aimed for one thing: distancing the sons of the God Emperor from a very stupid, costly, illegal, and immoral medical experiment carried out by the Japanese army. Nothing the Indonesians possessed could outweigh this strategic imperative. Anything or anybody was disposable in attaining it. The truth behind their mass murder of some nine hundred romusha was a threat to the thin illusion of friendly "big brother" occupation and could very possibly provoke the occupied Indonesians to rebellion. Mochtar and the Eijkman Institute became the Kenpeitai solution to the immediate political problem, and later as certain defeat materialized, his execution protected them from war tribunal justice.

Although the Kenpeitai convicted and sentenced Mochtar as early as January 1945, they would not execute him until early July. Mochtar's powerful friends, including the soon to be first vice president of Indonesia, the intellectual Mohammad Hatta, repeatedly pleaded with the Japanese to spare his life. The Japanese apparently carried out their execution of Mochtar only after finally realizing they had no prospect of a future in Indonesia. Why would they do so? What had they done at Klender that incited the murder of Mochtar as a necessity?

An understanding of both the mechanics and depth of immorality of this act begins with a look at the colonial Netherlands East Indies immediately prior to the invasion and occupation by Japan. Mochtar's role as a respected and accomplished scientist at the Eijkman Institute in Batavia placed both the man and the institute itself on the occupier's bloody execution ground. What did the Japanese occupiers sacrifice for their ill-gotten liberty? More to the lone bright point of this dark history: What did Mochtar sacrifice for the liberty of his colleagues?

FOUR

Netherlands East Indies

Colonial Rule

In 1938 rumors of war assailed Europe while China bled with actual war, but a sun-dappled optimism prevailed among the Dutch citizens of Batavia. In response to gloomy talk of war, they held extravagant galas to raise funds for the purchase of Spitfire fighter airplanes in defense of the homeland, Holland, against the suddenly turgid Nazi threat. They knew full well that a belligerent Japan was capable of attacking neighbors and that it aspired to reap the mineral wealth of their archipelago. Their own colonial forces, the Koninklijk Nederlands Indisch Leger (KNIL), were manned, trained, and equipped against internal rather than external threats. They certainly understood this fact but not the serious vulnerability it imposed. Instead, they felt securely positioned behind the more outward-looking colonial forces elsewhere in the region: American forces in the Philippines and British troops in the Federated Malay States. The nearby fortress of Singapore harbored the invincible British Royal Navy, a maritime force without peer in the South China Sea.

Their hold upon the East Indies seemed firm and unshakable, despite Japan's ruthless ambitions and the faint rumblings of nationalist sentiment among native Indonesians. Their steadfast social, political, and economic sovereignty over the islands, established over 320 years, had been interrupted only once. In 1811 the British invaded and conquered Java, then defended by Dutch and French troops. Sir Stamford Raffles (to found the city of Singapore in 1819) was appointed lieutenant governor general of Java (by Lord Minto, governor in India). Raffles and his wife, Olivia Mariamne, were to make an indelible mark on Java during their brief reign over it, including the discovery and excavation of the massive Buddhist Borobudur temple at Magelang in central Java and the abolition of slavery and the opium trade. Indonesians today drive on the lefthand side of the road by writ of Lieutenant Governor General Raffles.

Olivia perceived the Dutch residents of Java as being absorbed into Malay lifestyle and culture. They had broadly embraced Javanese clothing, diet, and a generally non-European lifestyle, including widespread and socially tolerated intermarriage with local women. She actively reversed the trend, affirming European dress, diet, manner, and unions for Europeans as the social norm in Java. In late 1814 Olivia died of cholera at Batavia, and her grave remains today in the old Tanah Abang cemetery in central Jakarta. A stirring monument to her erected by Raffles stands in the historic Botanical Gardens at Bogor south of Jakarta. Her loss devastated Raffles, and he returned to England in 1815 after the British handed the colony back to Holland (despite his strong protests). The colony had been bartered with the Anglo-Dutch treaty of 1814, signed in the wake of the Napoleonic wars. The British had no interest in having a new ally emasculated by the loss of its key source of wealth and power.

Despite the exit of the Raffles, the social walls erected between Europeans and Javanese held fast, and the Dutch thereafter on Java strived to retain their European identities against the siren sensibility and comfort of Javanese ways. Likewise, as European influence held fast among the colonizers, the Dutch discouraged adoption of European ways by "inlanders" or indigenous peoples. The racially defined master-servant tenor of colonial rule had been set for the century that followed.

Though the colonists would rule sternly and to their vast advantage, they would eventually begin liberalizing their reign over the islands. In some ways 1938 may be considered the zenith of Dutch colonial mastery of the East Indies. Profit margins for the rapacious voc (Vereenigde Oost-Indische Compagnie or United East Indies Company) and the Crown government had become much lower than during the first two centuries of their dominion. In 1938 income derived from the East Indies amounted to just 13.7 percent of Netherlands gross domestic product. Friend explains that businessmen and government officers at the time thought the contribution much higher, at around 40 to 50 percent. This in part explains their post-war slogan, *"Indies lost, disastrous cost."*[1] The colonists had been systematically reforming their rule in the direction of a still distant equity for Indonesians. The Dutch colonialists of 1938 participated in radical and broad reforms of their governance of the East Indies. They had begun aiming for wealth derived from the colony to build the colony rather than to increase the wealth of the motherland.

Colonial Reform

The Dutch had finally come around, though far too late, to the concept of building a colony suited to advancement of the colonized. Model cities like Bandung, as well as institutions of research and education, were at last being built. An indigenous (or imported) merchant class, though representing a small slice of the population, thrived and educated their children in their own superb schools. Cracks had appeared in the walls erected around the adoption of aspects of Dutch culture, as in language and education, by indigenous people. The rise of Dr. Abu Hanifah (to become Dutch naval medical officer, then revolutionary commander and first minister of education of the United States of Indonesia), documented in his autobiographical book, *Tales of a Revolution*, exemplifies this dramatic shift. His uncle, Professor Achmad Mochtar, represented a similarly rare and towering rise above the very hard ceilings imposed by Dutch colonial rule upon Indonesia's indigenous people. Indonesians finally began obtaining a share of the rewards that their rich homeland offered. An intellectual elite emerged in these reforms.

Such changes were coming quickly and furiously and reaching deeper than the indigenous elite alone. The Dutch had created a penal sanction law around 1900 that resulted in coolies being indentured for trivial violations of work contracts they could scarcely understand. Many thousands became, in effect, slaves to their contract holders. Haji Agus Salim, a prominent Indonesian Muslim leader of the early twentieth century, referred to these laws as "this stain on civilization, this blow in the face of humanity."[2] Although the Dutch parliament voted a renewal of the penal sanction in 1924, more sensible and progressive Dutch in the East Indies actively undermined its practices. Reform was in the air. On the east coast of Sumatra in 1929, for example, the ratio of indentured to free coolies was 261,000 to 40,813. In 1940 it was 53 to 215,670.[3] Indentured servitude was being actively eradicated. The cruel yoke of colonialism eased even among the Indonesian masses in this era.

Although a history dominated by the rise and aggression of Imperial Japan clearly demonstrated Dutch tardiness in their arrested progressive colonial thinking, the colonialists were nevertheless finally moving in an admirable direction. Even by the standards of racial equal opportunity today, some of the late initiatives by the Dutch appear truly remarkable.

An outstanding example of their evolving thinking in the early twentieth century may be found in the Eijkman Institute. That institution of medical research, in the Batavia of 1938, was a rare asset of worldwide significance in the rapidly maturing field of tropical medicine and hygiene. It was also rare ground where Dutch and Indonesian alike were judged and advanced according to merit rather than ethnicity or creed: an astonishingly level playing field in endeavors of advanced technology and importance. The investment of the Dutch in this enterprise was to generate a great stride forward in medical science. One example was the discovery of the cause, cure, and prevention of beriberi: vitamin B1. This led to the discovery of all vitamins and other micronutrients and vast improvements in the nutrition and health of all humanity.

Beriberi and the Eijkman Institute

Up until 1938 the Eijkman Institute was called Centraal Laboratorium van den Dienst der Volksgezondheid (Central Laboratory for Public Health). A photograph of the front of the institute taken in 1938 shows both names. This year was the fiftieth anniversary of the institute's founding by the distinguished Dutch researcher Christiaan Eijkman and the ninth anniversary of Eijkman being awarded the Nobel Prize for Physiology or Medicine.

Fifty-two years earlier, in 1886, Professor C. H. Pekelharing and Dr. C. Winkler were dispatched from Holland to investigate the serious problem of beriberi in workers, prisoners, and soldiers in the

East Indies. At this time the citadels of medical science in Europe were beginning to unravel the relationships between microorganisms and human diseases. Men like Robert Koch and Louis Pasteur led this charge, and by 1886 armies of scientists were at work on the problem. Pekelharing and Winkler came to Java bent upon finding the supposed microbial basis of beriberi. At this stage in medical progress, no one knew anything of micronutrients (vitamins and essential minerals). Christiaan Eijkman and his colleagues in Batavia were to initiate this revolutionary advance.

After Pekelharing and Winkler returned to Holland empty-handed with respect to a microbial culprit (in retrospect, a genuine credit to their conduct of science), they left behind Dr. Christiaan Eijkman, a student of Robert Koch, to carry on their search for the germ responsible for beriberi. In 1888 the governor general of the Netherlands East Indies appointed Eijkman as the director of the new research laboratory at the Central Military Hospital at Weltevreden (today Gatot Subroto Hospital of the Indonesian Army at Senen). This marked the beginning of what would become the Eijkman Institute in 1938.

Eijkman gradually abandoned the microbial search instigated by his distant masters. He turned his attention to diet after noticing a relationship between what was fed to chickens and a condition of polyneuritis that they sometimes contracted, a disease that resembled beriberi in humans. This may be one of the earliest examples of an animal model for a human disease, and Eijkman's thorough exploitation of it was brilliantly far ahead of his time.

Eijkman noted that his laboratory chickens no longer developed severe polyneuritis after the man tending them changed their diet. As a matter of economy, the caretaker had been feeding the chickens with polished rice left over from the military hospital kitchen. However, the managers of the hospital mess decided that they did not like the idea of civilian chickens enjoying their fine military rice, so they cut off the supply. The laboratory man had to revert to purchasing cheap unpolished rice for the birds. Soon after he initiated that change, the polyneuritis among the chickens vanished. Eijkman published these observations in 1890: polished rice as the cause of polyneuritis in chickens, and unpolished rice as its cure.

This random but keen observation opened the door for the greatest achievement of Eijkman's career and an enormous advance in medical science. Through carefully controlled pathology studies, he linked polyneuritis in chickens with beriberi in humans. Eijkman and his colleague G. Grijns went on to effectively rule out a bacteriological etiology for beriberi. On the basis of this evidence and their urging, unpolished red rice was introduced to prison meals in the East Indies, and highly prevalent beriberi among the inmates, as with polyneuritis in Eijkman's chickens, vanished as if by magic.

Chemists around the world began searching for the substance responsible for the elimination of beriberi in humans. More than two decades would pass before thiamine, or vitamin B1, would be purified and confirmed as that substance. Remarkably, the first successful crystalline pure preparation of vitamin B1 would come from chemists at the Eijkman Institute in Batavia. In 1926 B.C.P. Jansen and W. P. Donath, starting with 300kg of rice pericarp (a wispy material that must have been hugely voluminous), obtained less than one-hundredth of a gram of pure thiamine (vitamin B1). They sent milligram amounts to collaborators in Holland, including Eijkman himself, and in the United States to prove or disprove the hypothesis that this exceedingly miniscule quantity of a substance could explain such dramatic human health effects—a notion that evoked incredulity among most scientists of that era. The kilograms of proteins, carbohydrates, fats, and salts in the foods that we consume daily, it was reasoned, accounted for good health. The milligrams of thiamine sent from the Eijkman Institute would shatter that earnestly held belief.

The Dutch collaborated with R. R. Williams, who worked at Bell Telephone Laboratories in New Jersey. Williams had studied the beriberi problem in the Philippines in the 1900s and retained a key interest. He pursued it in his spare time with a modest grant from the Fleischmann Yeast Company. Williams and Eijkman each independently confirmed the identity of the crystal as the chemical responsible for the prevention and cure of polyneuritis in chickens. In 1926 they finally confirmed the "vitamin theory"—that specific molecules in seemingly infinitesimal quantities constituted indispensable elements of nutrition, the absence of which caused serious and even fatal human disease.[4] In 1929 Eijkman, by this time a longtime resident in Holland, was awarded the Nobel Prize for this discovery. He was too ill by then to travel to Stockholm to receive his prize, and he passed away a few months later.

Tropical Infections and the Eijkman Institute

The Eijkman Institute's research agenda also went into realms beyond nutrition. The burden of infectious diseases of the tropics was the primary motivator of research in tropical medicine. Indeed, even Eijkman's work started down the avenue of infections, and only good science diverted him to a problem of nutrition. The bulk of work at the institute engaged the full spectrum of tropical infectious diseases. This expansion of scope accelerated in 1916, when the institute moved from the old military hospital facility at Senen into the massive building at Salemba that it occupies to this day.

A review of the published contributions of the institute reveals names of great prominence in the very young field of tropical medicine: G. W. Kiewiet de Jonge, J. A. Boorsma, P. C. Flu, and E. W. Walch. In 1899 the institute hosted the great German pathologist Robert Koch for several months, during which time he conducted microscopic surveys of malaria on Java that led him to postulate a naturally acquired immunity to malaria. The entomology team in 1916 included the famous S. T. Darling. The contributions in anopheline mosquito biology, taxonomy, and malaria epidemiology (in collaboration with fellow Dutch scientists Schüffner, Swellengrebel, and many others) pioneered malariology in Asia, and their works remain widely cited today.

In the 1880s and 1890s, the state of tropical medicine in the rest of the world could be fairly described as so embryonic as to be almost useless. When the French initiated work on the Panama Canal in 1881, yellow fever and malaria killed them and their imported laborers en masse.[5] Their doctors' only advice against these grave threats, which of course was of no value, was for them to limit their consumption of fruit and to behave morally.

The heavy mortality due to tropical diseases at Panama forced the French to surrender their canal-building effort in 1888, precipitating scandal and collapse of the government in Paris. The vital role of mosquitoes in the diseases of the tropics was by then only just being dimly understood. Sir Patrick Manson, a Scottish physician scientist working at Hong Kong in the 1880s, had described the transmission of parasitic filarial worms by mosquitoes. By 1900 a fuller recognition had dawned with the work of Walter Reed on yellow fever in Cuba and that of Ronald Ross on malaria in India under remote guidance from Manson. William Gorgas applied this understanding to the American effort at the canal in Panama with spectacular success.

The economic and health dividends delivered at Panama by 1914 awakened tropical medicine and hygiene as a worthwhile human endeavor, that is, by the lights of early twentieth-century minds, one yielding enormous economic and strategic benefits. The British established schools that were wholly dedicated to tropical medicine and hygiene at London and Liverpool in the 1900s.[6] Physician scientist Ozwaldo Cruz helped established a serology institute in Brazil in 1900, which he turned into a tropical medicine research institute after becoming director in 1902. Individual scientists and physicians all around the developed world of this age began working in earnest on the diseases of the tropics within their broader institutions of health research.

The establishment of the laboratory headed by Eijkman in Batavia in 1888 can be considered the first serious scientific endeavor aimed directly at the diseases of the tropics. The Pasteur Institute at Bandung in western Java came in 1895. Through their investment of institutional capital in hygiene and tropical medicine, Dutch scientists on Java were several decades ahead of the rest of the world. They leveraged this investment against the rampant tropical infections surrounding them to reap huge health dividends in Indonesia and the region.

The 1938 yearbook for the Eijkman Institute lists the following fields of endeavor undertaken there: tropical physiology, tropical hygiene, pathology, anatomic pathology, and epidemiology (including beriberi, cholera, dysentery, leprosy, malaria, syphilis and other spirochetes, tuberculosis, typhus, filariasis, protozoa, intestinal helminthes, and meliodiosis), internal medicine, and medical entomology. No other institute of tropical medicine and hygiene in the world was as advanced and in such broad pursuit of scientific

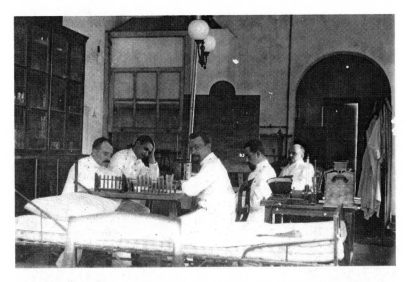

1. Dutch scientists at work in the public health laboratory embedded in the Central Military Hospital at Weltevreden, Batavia, ca. 1895. Published with the permission of the Royal Tropical Institute, Amsterdam.

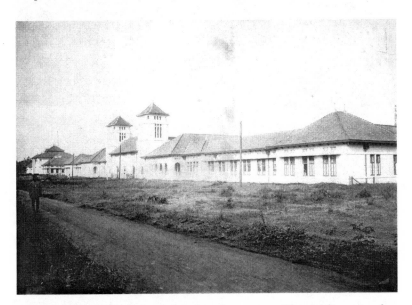

2. Central Hospital at Weltevreden, Batavia, ca. 1920. The stricken romusha from Klender were brought to this hospital and their tissues were examined at the Eijkman Institute, seen at far left of photo. Published with the permission of the Royal Tropical Institute, Amsterdam.

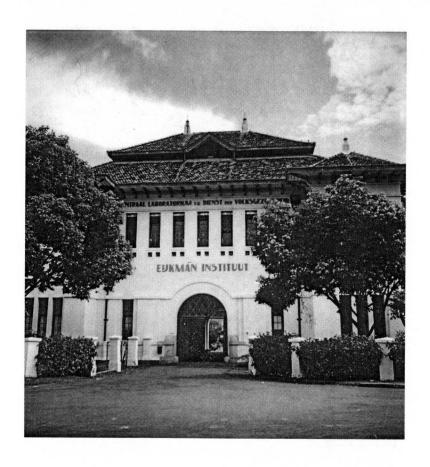

3. The Eijkman Institute in 1938. Published
with the permission of the Royal Tropical
Institute, Amsterdam.

4. (*Opposite*) Christiaan Eijkman, ca. 1925.
Published with the permission of the Royal
Tropical Institute, Amsterdam.

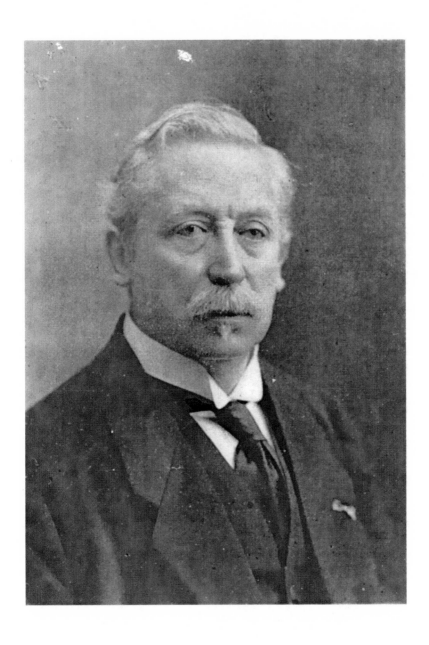

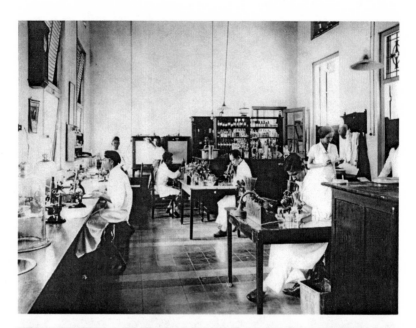

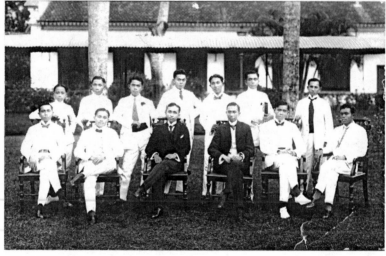

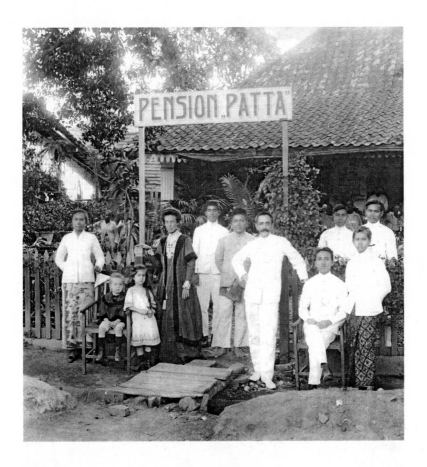

5. (*Opposite top*) The bacteriology laboratory in
the Eijkman Institute, ca. 1930. Published with
the permission of the Royal Tropical Institute,
Amsterdam.

6. (*Opposite bottom*) STOVIA graduates in May
1918. Marzoeki is seated second from left.
Dr. Aulia, who tended the stricken romusha at
Klender, is seated third from right. Published
with permission of Nita Dotulong Zahir, Jakarta.

7. (*Above*) Mochtar (*seated*) with the malaria
research team at Mandailing, Sumatra, ca.
1918. Published with the permission of Jolanda
van der Bom, Amsterdam.

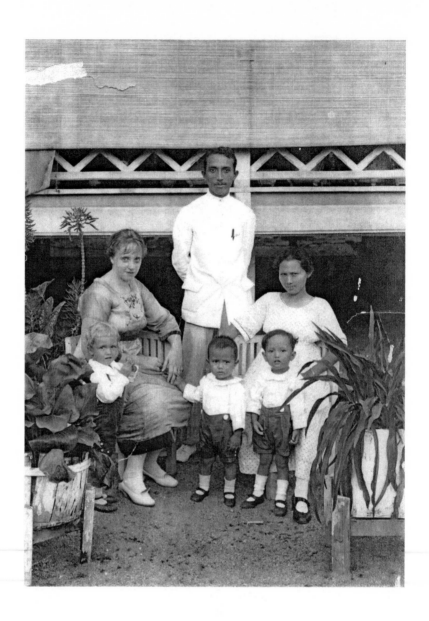

8. Mochtar and his family with a
Dutch woman and child at Mandailing,
ca. 1920. Published with the permission
of Jolanda van der Bom, Amsterdam.

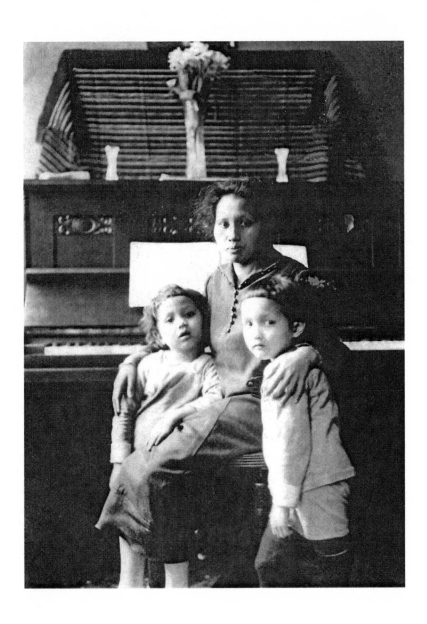

9. Siti Hasnah with Imramsjah and
Baharsjah in Amsterdam, ca. 1922.
Published with the permission of
Taty Hanafiah D. Uzar, Jakarta.

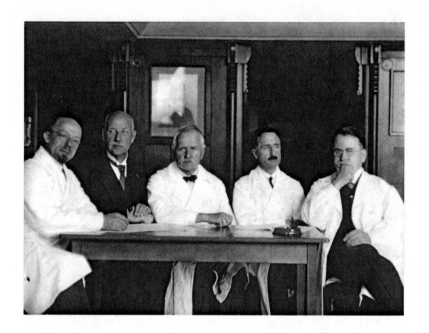

10. Mochtar's mentors Schüffner and Swellengrebel (*third and fourth from left*) with colleagues at the University of Amsterdam, ca. 1932. Published with the permission of the Royal Tropical Institute, Amsterdam.

11. (*Opposite*) Portrait of Achmad Mochtar as a young man, with his wife, Siti Hasnah, in 1927. Published with the permission of Jolanda van der Bom, Amsterdam.

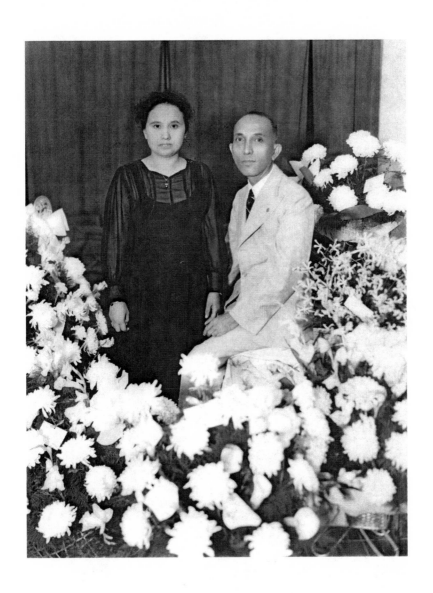

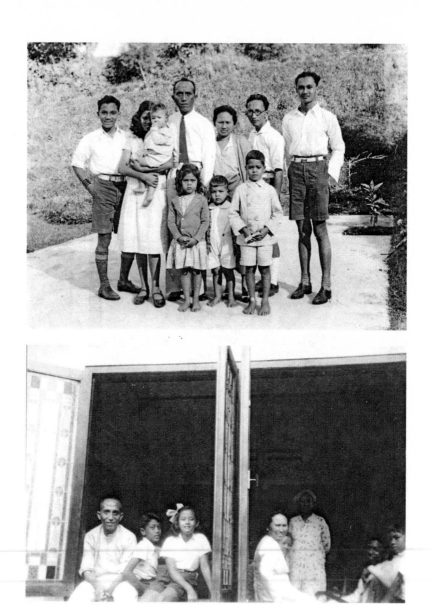

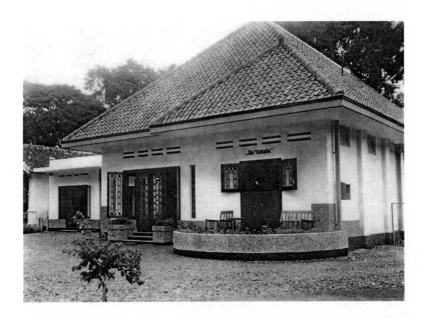

12. (*Opposite top*) Mochtar and Siti Hasnah with family
and relatives at Semarang, Central Java, ca. 1935.
Imramsjah is at far left rear, and Baharsjah is second
from right at rear. Published with the permission of Bas
Mochtar, London.

13. (*Opposite bottom*) The Mochtar and Hanafiah families
lounging at Hastarimba at Cikini in Batavia, ca. 1940.
From left to right: Mochtar, an unknown nephew,
Taty, Siti Hasnah, Siti Ramah, the wife of Hanafiah,
Hanafiah, and Asikin. Published with the permission of
Taty Hanafiah D. Uzar, Jakarta.

14. (*Above*) The Mochtar home, Hastarimba, at Jalan
Raden Saleh No. 48, Cikini, Batavia, ca. 1938. Published
with the permission of Taty Hanafiah D. Uzar, Jakarta.

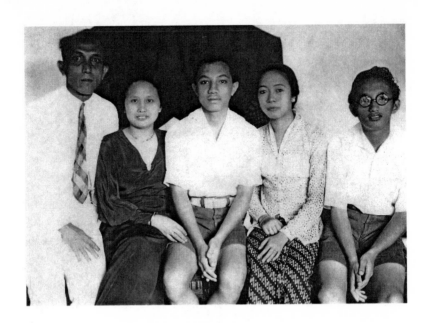

15. Mochtar with wife, sons, and Siti
Ramah, ca. 1934. Published with the
permission of Taty Hanafiah D. Uzar,
Jakarta.

16. (*Opposite*) Mochtar's sons, Baharsjah
(*left*) and Imramsjah, in Leiden with
Nazir Pamuntjak, ca. 1940. Published
with the permission of Taty Hanafiah
D. Uzar, Jakarta.

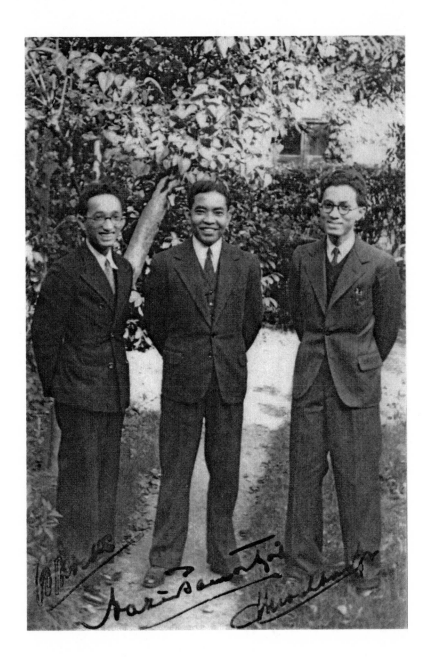

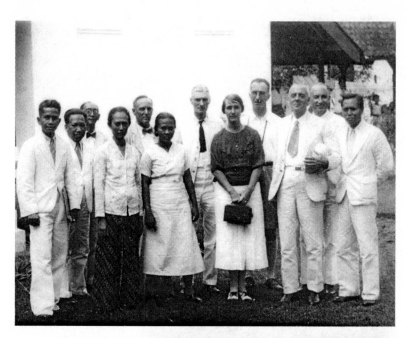

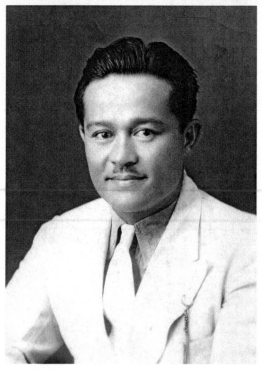

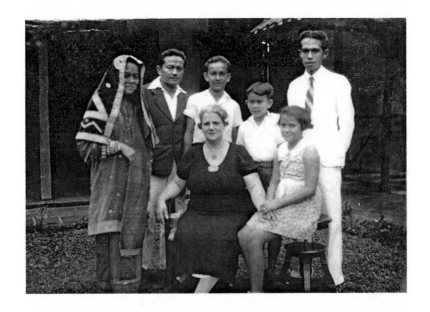

17. (*Opposite top*) Raden Soesilo (*far right*) hosting
malariologist Emilio Pampana (*fourth from right*) and
the delegation from the League of Nations Health
Organization, Sumatra, 1936. Soesilo was Mochtar's
STOVIA classmate, fellow doctoral student in Shuffner's
laboratory at the University of Amsterdam, and colleague
at the Eijkman Institute, where he headed the Malariology
Laboratory. In 1943 the Japanese beheaded Soesilo at
Banjarmasin, Borneo, after accusing him of meeting
American submarines at the Barito River. Published with
the permission of the Royal Tropical Institute, Amsterdam.

18. (*Opposite bottom*) Portrait of Dr. Marzoeki, Batavia,
ca. 1937. Published with the permission of Latifah Kodijat
Marzoeki, Jakarta.

19. (*Above*) Marzoeki family portrait, Sukabumi, Java,
1938. Corrie is seated center, with Latifah seated next to
her. Latifah's two brothers stand behind their mother, and
Marzoeki is in a dark jacket. The man and woman at right
and left are cousins. Published with the permission of
Latifah Kodijat Marzoeki, Jakarta.

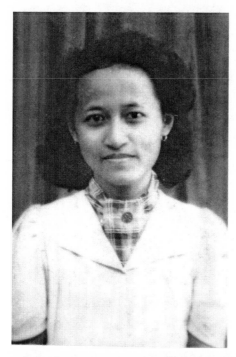

20. Nani Kusumasudjana, Batavia, ca. 1939. Published with the permission of Kantjana Gumira Kusuma Sudjana, Jakarta.

21. Staff of the Eijkman Institute, 1938. Mochtar is seated fourth from the right. Director Mertens is seated center, between two men. Published with the permission of the Royal Tropical Institute, Amsterdam.

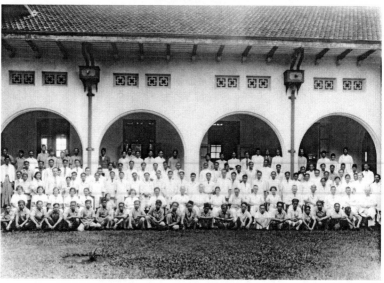

excellence and tropical public health impact across such a broad array of fields.

In Europe and America the new tropical medicine specialists generally remained based in their home countries, occasionally conducting sorties into the tropics. Many of the scientists at the Eijkman Institute, in contrast, had actually been born in the East Indies (like many of the colonialists of this era). The Dutch director, W. K. Mertens, was born at Surabaya in East Java. All of the Dutch staff members were, at the very least, long-term residents of Java.

Even more remarkably, and again without precedent anywhere else in this era, the Eijkman Institute had native Indonesian scientists functioning as fully contributing peer investigators. This trend in their staffing began in 1922, with the addition of Kadiroen and R. Soedarsono. By 1938 they had been joined by H. E. Latuasan, Klaasen, S. Kertoredjo, M. S. Sastrodarsono, M. Soedarsono, R. S. Adikkoesoemo, R. G. Pringgosoedirdjo, Soewarto, and Jatman (much more on the remarkable Mr. Jatman later in this history).

Raden Soesilo, head of the malaria laboratory at the Eijkman Institute since 1931, published prolifically on malaria control in the East Indies. We discovered a photograph of Soesilo heading an Indonesian delegation meeting in Sumatra in 1936 with a League of Nations team of malaria experts headed by the internationally famed malariologist Emilio Pampana. Soekarnen published on meliodiosis (a devastating bacterial infection), M. Sardjito on leptospires (another bacterial disease) and on dysentery, S. Bagindo on malaria epidemiology, M. Soerono on malaria, and W. Joedo on leptospirosis. Dr. Achmad Mochtar joined the Eijkman Institute in 1937 and worked on the bacterium causing Weil's disease and other leptospira bacteria. In light of the racial barriers of this time and place (as most places of that era), this was an amazingly progressive arrangement. The long-established school of medicine for young Indonesians at Batavia, STOVIA, had made these bright and well trained native physician scientists available.

Examples abound of the contributions of the entire staff of the Eijkman Institute, beyond Dr. Eijkman's obvious and well-recognized work. Kiewiet de Jonge developed and perfected curricula still used in the teaching of tropical medicine, derived from three-month courses he led at the institute each year from 1901 until his retirement in 1914. De Haan in 1911 provided bacteriological evidence of the etiology of plague in Java, following up on the discovery of the bacterium *Yersinia pestis* by Yersin in Hong Kong and Vietnam. Lou Otten at Malang in 1913 conducted pioneering work on plague epidemiology. Otten went on to become director of the Pasteur Institute in Bandung, and he developed the vaccine against plague that brought the disease under control on Java by 1939. Moreover, Otten oversaw the production of cholera, smallpox, rabies, typhoid, and typhus vaccines at that institute, which were used on a massive scale in the East Indies as well as in Malaya, Vietnam, Thailand, and the Philippines before World War II. Otten's physician scientist wife, Maria J. Otten–van Stockum, conducted pioneering work in rabies vaccination.[7] Dutch colonial mastery in tropical medicine and hygiene was paying enormous health dividends throughout the region.

Otten's method for making heat-stable smallpox vaccine would go on to play an important role in the eventual eradication of the disease in 1980. Otten's institute also produced tetanus antitoxin, a plasma product derived by injecting horses with small amounts of tetanus toxin.

In the 1920s, the appointment of Brug as director of the Eijkman Institute saw greater emphasis placed on entomology and parasitology. Discovery of the important filarial worm parasite *Brugia malayi* (the cause of the horribly disfiguring disease called elephantiasis) and its mosquito carriers came directly from the work of Brug and DeRook. Brug brought mosquito taxonomy and systematics to the study of endemic mosquito-borne diseases in the East Indies. Walch, Soesilo, von Hell, and Bonne-Wepster collectively pioneered this exhaustive work among the two dozen species of malaria-carrying anopheline mosquito varieties occurring along the length of the archipelago. In so doing they brought mosquito species identity into the realms of science and public health—work that remains an essential element of tropical medicine and hygiene.

In Sumatra, Mertens conducted some of the first epidemiological studies of dengue fever. Mertens and van Veen unraveled the mysterious cause of "bongkrek" poisoning as a bacillus contaminating the fungal fermentation of coconuts with the toxins toxoflavine and bongkrek acid. Mertens also isolated leptospire bacteria from wild cats, identifying them as important reservoirs of human infection.

Mochtar and his colleagues at the Eijkman Institute and their many partners made important and lasting contributions to the field of tropical medicine and hygiene. We strive to affirm this fact in setting the stage for grasp of the weight of the crime of destroying the institute in 1945.

Tropical Medicine and Hygiene

In contemporary tropical medicine and hygiene, the early accomplishments of the Eijkman Institute researchers and their colleagues around the archipelago tend to be overshadowed by those of other pioneers of the field like Manson, Ross, Gorgas, Reed, Christophers, Watson, Soper, and others so dominant in the English medical literature of the time. This is in part a product of the almost complete dominance of English as the preferred language of science today, a condition that began in earnest only after World War II. In today's scientific community, technical articles published in any language but English border upon international irrelevance and tend to be largely ignored outside of the countries where they are published.

The community of science seems to carry this language bias today even as it looks to the past. It would be an error of arrogance or laziness to extrapolate the lesser importance of non-English publications today to the very dawn of biomedical scientific endeavor. Early scientists published critically important papers in French, German, Dutch, Spanish, Italian, Portuguese, Russian, and Japanese, with no assigned notion of the preeminence of English for works of international importance. This was certainly true at the Eijkman Institute of the 1930s, the world's leader in tropical medicine and hygiene. Papers from that period, virtually all in Dutch, reflect pioneering work in tropical medicine that today remains linguistically inaccessible to the majority of scientists in that field. Nonetheless, the richness of work in tropical medicine and hygiene conducted by the Eijkman Institute and their collaborators had few peers in the 1930s. The institute was also many decades ahead on breaking down the racial barriers to scientific advancement.

The field of tropical medicine and hygiene today remains a humanitarian effort, largely focused upon infections endemic to developing nations throughout the tropics. Scientists committed to this field labor to bring new human knowledge and technology to bear upon the enormous disease burdens still imposed by tuberculosis, malaria, dysentery, and HIV, along with diseases like leptospirosis, dengue fever, and leishmaniasis. The dominance of developed nations in science translates to those endeavors. Consequently, scientists working in North American and European laboratories have contributed the most in tropical medicine and hygiene over the past six decades. As recently as 1980, only a handful of substantial medical research laboratories operated permanently in the tropics, the majority of them run by the American military or the network of laboratories of the Pasteur Institute (an enterprise of the French since 1887). The laboratories of developing nations, like those in Brazil, India, Malaysia, and the Philippines, struggled with limited resources and access to cutting-edge technology.

American armed forces learned the strategic importance of tropical diseases during the Pacific War. The U.S. Naval Medical Research Unit No. 2 was created on newly liberated Guam in 1944, later relocating to Taiwan (until 1979), the Philippines (until 1993), Indonesia (until 2010), and Singapore and Cambodia (until today). Its sister laboratory at Cairo (U.S. NAMRU-3) opened in 1946 and continues operating in 2014. Another laboratory at Lima, Peru (U.S. NAMRU-6), has operated since 1986. These laboratories conduct research on tropical infections of importance to their host countries and to militaries (principally malaria, mosquito-borne viruses, and enteric diseases).

Imported American investigators staffed most of these military labs. The host countries had relatively few scientists to offer, but efforts were made to train up local young scientists in these countries, and their efforts have borne real fruit. Likewise, the Oxford University Tropical Network, funded largely by the Wellcome Trust, today operates tropical medicine and hygiene laboratories in Kenya, Thailand, Vietnam, and Indonesia. Though American, British, and French investigators (and other nationalities) certainly abound at these facilities in the tropics, they work side by side with local investigators who may rightfully be considered peers of the foreign scientists. By 2014 these models had at last begun to resemble—in terms of effective encouragement, development, and use of native-born scientific talent—what the Eijkman Institute had already achieved a century earlier.

The crucial key to this unique accomplishment and arrangement was not only progressive racial thinking by the Dutch but also the very substantial investment made in educating native Indonesian physician investigators beginning in 1854. In so doing, the Dutch had been able to understand long before other Europeans and the Americans that scientific endeavor and success was by no means the exclusive domain of a single economically endowed race. By contrast, latent African American scientific talent in the United States would not be truly socially enabled and emergent until after the racial upheaval and legal reforms of the 1960s.

The Eijkman Institute of the 1930s was a remarkable beacon of racial and social justice. It was a concrete asset in the broad march of human progress against both illness and racial injustice, and the Dutch of that time and place deserve accolades for its visionary realization. It is a tragic irony that the Dutch also played a hand in the destruction of the Eijkman Institute, as will be explained in later chapters.

Dr. Mochtar, Batavia, 1938

The 1938 yearbook of the Eijkman Institute shows that its staff of twenty-eight investigators/ scientists published ten papers in peer-reviewed journals of medicine, chemistry, and public health in 1937. The reporting scientists included A. Mochtar, A. G. van Veen, R. Soesilo, J. C. Lanzing, J. K. Baars, C. van der Poel, Wisnoe Joedo, J. Bonne-Wepster, and S. L. Brug.

In this remarkable year, 127 scientists, technicians, administrators, secretaries, and maintenance staff gathered for a photograph in the courtyard. The arrangement of staff reflects seniority. The maintenance staff are kneeling or squatting on the ground in the front. Mid-level staff members stand at the side and the back. In the center, seated along a row stretching the length of the photo, are the senior scientists, with the director, Mertens, center right. Dr. Mochtar is seated in this row, fourth from the left. This group of people, their close collaborators, and all of their predecessors at this point represented the greatest scientific capital ever gathered in the tropics in the pursuit of practical knowledge in tropical medicine and hygiene.

Only a few portraits of Achmad Mochtar survive. One of them shows him in early middle age, probably around 1927, when he completed his doctoral work at the University of Amsterdam (fig. 11). He was then thirty-five years old, dressed neatly in a fine European suit with white cotton shirt and tie. His wife, Siti Hasnah, stands next to him. She is the older sister of his close friend and colleague, Dr. Ali Hanafiah (also related to Mochtar's nephew, Dr. Abu Hanifah, author of *Tales of a Revolution*). The couple look squarely into the camera. The pose, gaze, and countenance of Dr. Mochtar are those of a confident, accomplished man. The subtle smile of his wife seems to affirm this. She glows in his success. They have two small boys at home, Baharsjah and Imramsjah. Another photo, taken when the family resided in Amsterdam, shows the boys with their mother at her treasured piano (fig. 9).

Mochtar returned triumphantly to the Netherlands East Indies in 1927. We know from the record of his published papers that he took up residence in Bengkulu, West Sumatra, and then at Semarang, Central Java. At Semarang he began collaborations with Indonesian scientists at the Eijkman Institute, and by 1937 he joined them there.

We know a great deal about Mochtar at this time, largely thanks to the documentation and memory of the children of Dr. Ali Hanafiah: Dr. Asikin Hanafiah, who was born in 1932, and Mrs. Taty Delma Juzar, born in 1929. A visit with them in Jakarta in 2010 provided a wealth of information as well as many of the photographs of Mochtar illustrating this work.

The two families were very close, even though the Hanafiahs lived in Tangerang, about ten miles outside of Batavia. The Mochtars lived at Jalan Raden Saleh No. 48, in the Cikini neighborhood not far from the institute. The house was still there in 2014 (across the street from the locally famous Oasis Restaurant known for its Dutch Indies cuisine and serving style), but the home was in use as a place of business. Taty recalled that the families would take turns visiting one another on weekends. When at the Mochtar household, they would all pile into Mochtar's two cars and drive to the Glodok neighborhood of old Batavia to enjoy leisurely dinners of Chinese food. A photograph of one of these weekend visits survives: Dr. Ali Hanafiah titled it "Sunday at Tangerang," and it shows the two families lounging on the veranda of the Hanafiah home. Likewise, a picture of the families gathered at the house on Raden Saleh survives. The house is named Hastarimba, for Siti Hasnah, Mochtar, Imramsjah, and Baharsjah (fig. 14). The wife's name comes first in the matrilineal tradition of the Minangkabau of Indonesia, in which both Mochtar and his wife were born and raised. It is her house. She would have left it to a daughter, but none came.

Another photo shows Mochtar seated with his wife, two teenaged sons, and a cousin of Siti Hasnah, Siti Ramah (mother of famed Indonesian batik artist Irwan Tirta). This photo likely dates from 1937 (fig. 15).

Taty and Asikin recalled visiting the Mochtar household at a time when the two Mochtar boys were already in medical school in Holland. Asikin remembered being mothered by his aunt and receiving fatherly advice from his uncle. The house had a grand piano (not the upright that sufficed in Amsterdam), and Mrs. Mochtar loved playing it. She favored the classics, especially Mozart. Taty and Asikin recalled her reading books at every spare moment and of her running a very orderly household with a strict manner. She brooked no disobedience from Asikin. Taty and Asikin each referred to the house at Raden Saleh as "Pavilion," and remembered a constant stream of visiting family and students. A photograph from early 1941 shows the Mochtar and Hanafiah clans gathered at Hastarimba, with Taty and a cousin next to Mochtar in the window. Asikin sits in the right corner. In that photograph we see Mochtar the family man, at ease surrounded by those closest to him (fig. 13).

The Japanese would seize this house upon the occupation. The family retreated to another house nearby at Jalan Cikini Raya, across the street from a large school. The school still stands and remains in use as such, but the house is gone. Taty remembered the house as large and accommodating. She believed the Japanese had taken Hastarimba for its proximity and direct access to Cikini Hospital, directly behind it. The big house at Cikini Raya became a wartime refuge for Dr. Ali Hanafiah and his family, as well as for Dr. Abu Hanifah and his family.

The Mochtars were people of substantial financial means and generosity, especially with family and students of science and medicine. Taty and Asikin had no understanding of its source, but believed that their uncle was well paid by the institute. While still at Hastarimba, Mochtar perhaps managed patients at Cikini Hospital. Taty remembered a door at the rear wall of Hastarimba that opened directly onto the hospital compound.

A photo of the Mochtar boys from Taty and Asikin shows them in Holland, where they attended medical school, probably from 1940 (fig. 16). The man between them is Nazir Pamuntjak. The three of them lived in the same house in Leiden (Rijnsburgerweg 147; it still stood in 2011). Nazir at this time was about to complete his law degree and very likely took responsibility for getting the Mochtar boys settled and well behaved. He was already a nationalist leader and a close associate of Mohammad Hatta. The two had been arrested and jailed together in Amsterdam in the late 1920s, accused of plotting rebellion. Though no record survives, it also seems likely that Mochtar and Hatta would have been acquainted in Holland in the prior decade, though Hatta attended Erasmus University in Rotterdam during Mochtar's years at the University of Amsterdam.

Nazir went on to become Indonesia's ambassador to France. With Soekarno, Mohammad Hatta would give birth to the Republic of Indonesia after months of efforts at trying to save his friend, Professor Mochtar.

Mochtar and Siti Hasnah spent their energies doting on nieces and nephews at Hastarimba. They must have been proud of their distant and professionally maturing sons and relishing their highly promising futures. A photo of the couple from this period shows the gently aging Mochtar and a very happy Siti Hasnah.

We know that Mochtar in the period of 1927 to 1942 had a vibrant home, surrounded by loving family and the trappings of financial, professional, and intellectual success. He was an internationally recognized expert on leptospirosis and was surrounded by highly accomplished Indonesian and Dutch colleagues at the Eijkman Institute. In a group photo taken at a social gathering in 1940, Mochtar and Siti Hasnah are seen within the network of people closest to them, including several of the people later caught up in the Mochtar affair.

The occasion of the photo is not known, but in it we may glimpse the vibrant social dimension of the life they shared. In the collections of such photos owned by relatives and close associates, Mochtar and Siti Hasnah appear again and again.

Life had richly rewarded Mochtar's dedication and hard work, to both his family and his career. In the upcoming two chapters we will examine how Mochtar arrived at this enviable destination. His rise occurred within the institutions and events, and among the networks of people, that gave direct rise to the Republic of Indonesia.

FIVE

Coming of Age

The Minangkabau

Sumatra's nine hundred miles of volcanic mountains rise sharply out of the abyss of the stormy Indian Ocean, forming its westward face. East of the long ridge, the island slopes nearly two hundred miles and dissolves into the shallow Malacca Straits and Java Sea. Both ends of this island offer testimony of a restless and malleable Earth and of the impermanence of life—the Asian tsunami of 2004 at the far north, and the 1883 explosive disintegration of Mount Krakatoa in the far south. But these seemingly profound disasters were modestly gentle events compared to a day seventy thousand years ago when the super volcano at what is today Lake Toba in Sumatra erupted in a truly cataclysmic blast that dramatically changed the world's climate. Some scientists believe those effects provided a decisive survival advantage for intelligence that launched the dominance of modern humans. Twenty or thirty thousand years later the intrepid humans expanding out of Africa would reach Sumatra.

At the time of Mochtar's 1892 birth, tropical jungle still covered much of the immense island, harboring an abundance of tigers, leopards, elephants, rhinos, and orangutans. Sumatra's extraordinary beauty, biological diversity, and geological spasms mirror all of Indonesia and its history of riches, human diversity, wars, and sociopolitical landscapes altered by upheavals.

The hamlet of Mochtar's birth, Bonjol, sits directly on the equatorial line as it transects the western slopes of Sumatra's spine, in the middle of the island. Bonjol lies well above the steamiest jungles and enjoys a reasonably temperate climate. Coffee thrives on many small plantations. People live quiet and relatively prosperous agrarian lives. Padang cuisine, named for the capital city of the region, is popular all across Indonesia. This culinary tradition produced *rendang*, the spicy coconut-stewed beef that is synonymous with Indonesian cookery.

Rendang emerged from the kitchens of an ethnic group known as the Minangkabau, whose name translates as "victorious buffalo." Folklore explains that a powerful neighboring prince once challenged the Minangkabau people militarily. After negotiation, it was decided that a fight between two water buffalo would settle the dispute. At the appointed paddock and hour, the confident prince produced a massive, agitated bull with enormous sharp horns. The Minangkabau fielded, to the amusement of the prince, a mere calf for the battle. But its horns had been honed to razor sharpness, and it had been denied nourishment of any sort for several days. The little calf attracted no attention from the enormous buffalo, but it immediately raced to the bull. In its ravenous hunger the calf charged the bull's underside where it desperately poked and prodded in search of an udder. The calf sliced open the bull's belly, and it fell over mortally wounded. The invading prince had been outwitted.

The emphasis of this lore on triumph of the intellect over brawn permeates Minangkabau character. The rooflines of traditional Minangkabau homes, rising to sharp points at both ends, are a tribute to the victorious little buffalo—a constant reminder of their identity, its origins, and its lessons. Intellectual pursuits and development are the key to individual and group success.

Islam had not yet taken wide hold in the Indonesian archipelago in the 1500s. In the middle of that century, the already deeply Islamic Aceh sultanate at the northern tip of Sumatra invaded the animist Minangkabau, seizing their rich gold holdings and deposits. A century later, unhappy Minangkabau cut a deal with the Dutch at Batavia to evict the occupiers from Aceh in exchange for trading concessions. But many Minangkabau had by then adopted the deep Islam brought by the Acehnese. The Acehnese ultimately departed, but their rigid practice of the religion stayed among a faction of the Minangkabau. They called themselves the Padri and later campaigned widely and violently among neighboring Sumatran peoples, demanding strict adherence to their Wahabi-inspired form of Islam. They encountered stiff resistance. By the early 1800s they had been pushed back into their Minangkabau realm where traditional, elite syncretic groups opposed their assertion of dominance. A civil war ensued.

In 1815 the Padri murdered most of the Minangkabau royal family and forced capitulation of all Minangkabau to their rule. However, in 1821 the Dutch rallied the syncretic Minangkabau, and together they attacked the Padri, led by Imam Bonjol. An eleven-year war ensued that ended in defeat for the Padri. Divided and wounded by decades of wars, the Minangkabau people sought reconciliation of their animist traditions with their Islamic faith in order to avoid such devastating conflicts. The compromises melded Islam with distinct elements of their pre-Islamic traditions.

One of the most striking facets of Minangkabau life is its deeply matrilineal tradition (probably the largest such culture in existence today, with some 4 million adherents). Home and property are owned by the mother and passed to daughters. The men come and go from such households over the generations, while the female core of the clan remains constant. This creates a natural and encouraged stream that leads men away from the home. Around age seven they take up residence in local schools. Then, as teenagers, they leave the area in order to gather external wisdom for their people. Finally they return home to marry into the family and household of the wife's mother. Minangkabau men possess the hard cultural wiring for study and accomplishment in wholly unfamiliar surroundings.

This heritage largely explains the disproportionate representation of their men as leaders in the medicine, politics, arts, and commerce of Indonesia. They are a singularly industrious and successful ethnic group among Indonesia's many hundreds of other ethnic identities.

Colonial Education

Early in the twentieth century, higher education among natives was extremely rare in the Netherlands East Indies. In 1916 and 1917, only fifty-five students in all of the territories received certificates of completing a high school education. There were no universities of general education.

The Dutch of this period carefully controlled intellectual development. They feared and suppressed intellectual-driven nationalist sentiments of any stripe: communist, Islamist, royalist, or democratic
(all were present). They had no plan or intent for disengagement
from the islands—they were there to stay forever and strategized to
do so by restricting higher education to a select and manageable few.

The intellectual nationalist Mohammad Hatta, a Minangkabau,
would go on to demonstrate the reasoned basis of Dutch aversion to
indigenous intellectual development—it tended to expose the intrinsic injustice of colonial imperialism. Seeing Hatta's well-reasoned
and dispassionate persuasiveness on nationalism as misguided and
risky, the Dutch first imprisoned Hatta in Holland. Later freed and
undaunted, he persisted in his voice of reason and liberty, causing
the Dutch to exile him to the notoriously unhealthy Boven Digul
camp in the dark malarious swamps of remote Dutch New Guinea
(where many prisoners would die). Hatta would survive these ordeals
and go on to provide essential intellectual balance to the charismatic
Javanese firebrand Soekarno in birthing the Republic of Indonesia in 1945. The acknowledged importance of the pair rather than
Soekarno alone is expressed in the name of Jakarta's main airport
today, Soekarno-Hatta International. Large statues of the two men—
Soekarno holding a baton, and Hatta a thick book—greet visitors
driving onto that facility. Their statues also adorn the site in Jakarta
of Indonesia's proclamation of independence on August 17, 1945,
at Menteng in central Jakarta (not far from where Barack Obama
attended grade school in the late 1960s).

The Dutch view on education was not necessarily aimed solely at
its colonial possessions. Friend contrasts education in the Netherlands with the United States: the proportion of teenagers in school
in 1938 was 40 and 70 percent, respectively. This societal stance
was reflected in their colonial possessions; in 1938, 10.7 percent
of the total population of the American-administered Philippines
were enrolled in school, compared to just 3.2 percent of the Netherlands East Indies (and even this paltry proportion represented a
vast improvement relative to 1920).[1] Such discrepancies were even
greater at levels of higher education. Friend writes,

The American system of education was clearly oriented toward the mass, while the structure of education in the Netherlands, like that in most of Europe, ". . . had the effect of reinforcing class distinctions and reducing the flow of social mobility . . . the upper levels of education were the preserve of the upper classes." [J. E. Talbott, *The History of Education*, Daedalus 1971, 136.] Those who squeezed through the Dutch universities, however, were usually grounded in the classics, fluent in two or more Western languages, well-spoken in their own tongue, and familiar with other subjects of consequence.[2]

He goes on to say, "All figures illustrate the fact that Americans concentrated on 'education for citizenship' and made sacrifices for the sake of quantity, whereas the Dutch considered a few persons 'educated to perfection' to be a significant and satisfactory achievement." Thus the educational elitism of the Dutch in their colonies reflected their broader values as a society rather than a strictly colonial arrogance or cruelty aimed at other races or subordinated peoples.

The Dutch indeed opened, just barely, the doors of its higher educational system to the elite native sons and, all the more remarkably, daughters of Netherlands East Indies. A 1926 photo of Indonesian students at Utrecht University in the Netherlands celebrating the end of Ramadan illustrates this. We see nine students, three of them women, dressed as ladies and gentlemen smiling confidently at the camera (one of the gentlemen being the grandfather of Sangkot Marzuki, coauthor of this book).

The STOVIA Crucible

Higher education in medicine was another matter in the East Indies. In this field alone the Dutch acted deliberately—educating these specialists with superb training and in substantial numbers. Physicians were hugely useful in the Netherlands East Indies. Malaria was rampant in Batavia and almost everywhere else, along with typhoid, scrub typhus, plague, Weil's disease (leptospirosis), filariasis, leprosy, beriberi, and many other afflictions common in the Asian tropics. There could be no overabundance of doctors to deal with these serious challenges.

In 1854 a Dr. Bosch had the idea to enlist locally trained health workers to help cope with a disease outbreak at Banyumas, Java, by teaching them to administer vaccinations. This training program quickly expanded into something very much resembling a medical education at the Dutch military hospital at Weltevreden (Senen) in Batavia. Christiaan Eijkman and his laboratory were formally attached to this school from 1888 to 1896. In 1898 the facility was acknowledged as a medical school and dubbed the School tot Opleiding Van Inlandsche Artsen (School of Education for Native Doctors), or STOVIA.

A huge campus (15,742 square meters) for STOVIA was constructed near the military hospital and opened in 1902. Achmad Mochtar received his medical education there. Admission was tough, and the academics were grueling. The school produced superb physicians and intellectuals. At a time when annual high school graduates in all of the East Indies amounted to just a few dozen, STOVIA by 1927 had graduated 551 physicians. The most intellectually hungry of the indigenous young from all corners of the vast colony gravitated to medicine as practically the only door to higher learning of any kind. The best and brightest of the Indonesian archipelago landed at STOVIA, and these young people came to define themselves as a group. In so doing they deliberately brought definition to the very notion of being "Indonesian."

Out of necessity, the Dutch doctors running STOVIA in the early days accepted students lacking high school diplomas—none having those were to be found. They solved this problem by building into the curriculum three years of preliminary education in mathematics, languages (Dutch and German were required), and other subjects to prepare the students for the barrages of zoology, botany, chemistry, physics, anatomy, physiology, histology, and pathology that would form the core of their medical education of seven years. In total it was a grueling ten-year curriculum, with students required to live at STOVIA for the duration. Most of them arrived, as we believe Achmad Mochtar did in 1906, around the tender age of fourteen. We know with certainty that he was born in 1892 and graduated from STOVIA on June 21, 1916.

A photo of the entire STOVIA student body and teachers from 1916 includes mere boys. They are wearing short pants, most squatting in front or scattered along the sides. The upperclassmen wear long pants and jackets and stand toward the rear. Mochtar stands among them. Four girls are seen in the row behind the seated Dutch professors. STOVIA, in effect, raised these boys and girls. The students would come to know and view one another, in an emotional sense, as perhaps more like family than their biological kin at distant homes.

During Mochtar's time there as a junior student, senior students at STOVIA grasped an important idea and turned it into a guiding principle of nationality. Though they came from dozens of distinct cultures scattered among the far-flung islands, speaking different mother languages and observing many religious traditions, they were united across several fronts besides their medical training. They could speak to one another in a common, improvised language, though it was not the mother tongue of any of them.[3] More important, they preferred using that language over the fluent Dutch that got them through admissions to STOVIA and its curriculum. They resented Dutch dominance in governance and the economy, and they rejected notions of the racial superiority of the whites. These bright young people conceived of their scattered islands, languages, religions, and cultures as a unifiable whole. On May 20, 1908, nine students meeting in the anatomy classroom at STOVIA formed Boedi Oetomo (Utmost Ideal), an organization chartered to promote education but which evolved into the intellectual blueprint for the Republic of Indonesia. That classroom symbolizes for Indonesians what Independence Hall in Philadelphia inspires for Americans, though the Indonesian declaration of independence would only come thirty-seven years later at a site a few blocks from the Eijkman Institute.

Boedi Oetomo had initially been an exclusively aristocratic Javanese enterprise, but a young Javanese doctor named Tjipto Mangoengkoesoemo soon opened the society to working classes and those beyond Java. It evolved into a political movement. The massive hospital complex next door to the modern Eijkman Institute is named after him and known widely as "Cipto Hospital."[4]

In 1928 STOVIA students and others from the school of law (their school would later become the Kenpeitai headquarters and prison in

Jakarta) convened a Boedi Oetomo–inspired congress of youth from all across the Netherlands East Indies at a meeting hall at Kramat in Batavia. Mochtar's nephew, Abu Hanifah, a STOVIA student, was among the lead organizers. Those present formulated the Soempah Pemoeda, or Youth Pledge. This is how it reads:

> Firstly, we the sons and daughters of Indonesia acknowledge one motherland, Indonesia. Secondly, we the sons and daughters of Indonesia acknowledge one nation, the nation of Indonesia. Thirdly, we the sons and daughters of Indonesia uphold the language of unity, Indonesian.

The building where they recited this pledge stands today as a monument on the western side of a crowded major artery of Jakarta, Jalan Kramat at Senen. The expression of Indonesian language as a uniting entity is a key element of Indonesian identity to the present day. It remains effectively a second language for a vast majority of Indonesians representing hundreds of mother tongues among them. Bahasa Indonesia was declared a formal language upon independence in 1945, and it is the language of national education, media, commerce, and law.

That the idea for a great nation was hatched by a small group of men all under twenty-four years of age defies imagination. Yet twenty years later, their concept of a unified Indonesia gelled in the minds of the next generation, as expressed in the Youth Pledge. A generation later, it became reality. Today a restored STOVIA building in Senen is the Museum of the History of the National Awakening.

The men and women of STOVIA had an extraordinary camaraderie that would endure. Their bond was professional, personal, and political, like a very large and closely integrated family. They protected, promoted, and married one another. They treated one another's families without thought of fees. Most of the people mentioned in this history led lives in the heavy orbit of STOVIA.

Though this is pure speculation, one cannot help but see this profound blurring of family and professional lines in the ultimate sacrifice made by Mochtar in late 1944. He acted not just on behalf of his co-workers and subordinates, but also to save people he would have viewed very much as family.

In 1921 STOVIA relocated to the building in the Salemba neigh-borhood of Jakarta that it occupies today (as the Faculty of Medicine, University of Indonesia), near the Eijkman Institute. The inherent elitism of Dutch education, as expressed in the East Indies of the 1900s, created the STOVIA crucible, focusing the flower of intellect of an entire nation into a single professional field and onto a single campus. Medicine and intellectual politics married at STOVIA, and its doctors would go on to play leadership roles in the political future of the East Indies and, later, the bloody forging of their republic. Ali Hanafiah lists the names of seventeen STOVIA doctors lost in the war for independence against the Dutch (1945-49).[5]

The founding leader of Boedi Oetomo, STOVIA student Soetomo, was the older brother of Raden Soesilo, Mochtar's fellow PhD stu-dent in Amsterdam under W.A.P. Schüffner and later his colleague at the Eijkman Institute. The Japanese would behead Soesilo (at Ban-jarmasin, Borneo, December 1943) after accusing him of plotting against them. His alleged offense seems as unlikely as Mochtar's: exchanging messages with American submarines lurking in the Barito River of eastern Borneo. The Japanese viewed STOVIA men and women, with good justification, as reasoned and intelligent (and therefore dangerous) political thinkers. They were fated to suffer ter-ribly for this assessment during the occupation. The Japanese exe-cuted at least 19 STOVIA doctors.

The fact that STOVIA was an incubator of political thought and action was not lost on the Japanese occupiers. A haunting Japanese propaganda film shows the "opening" of the school of medicine (renamed Ika Dai Gaku) with pomp and ceremony in 1943. High-level Japanese officers are shown arriving and students and faculty in mil-itary parade bowing before them.[6] A Japanese rector was appointed, and Achmad Mochtar became the vice rector. A photograph taken shortly before the deaths at Klender in 1944 shows the "faculty" of Ika Dai Gaku, with Mochtar the lone Indonesian seated among uni-formed, sword-bearing medical men of the Japanese army (fig. 24). The Japanese army firmly controlled the medical school and its dan-gerously bright and proud students.

Soekarno's autobiography describes an incident involving medical students at that campus soon after the Japanese took over in 1943:

When the Japanese began controlling their curriculum, they rebelled. To instigate punishment, the Japanese shaved the tops of the students' heads and beat their bald spots with the full force of a heavy ruler. The students went out on strike. They were immediately jailed. For three months they were tortured, then sentenced to death.[7]

He goes on to describe how he pleaded with the Japanese to spare the students, which they did.

Mochtar's role in that event is described in a book on the history of the birth of Indonesia.[8] When the students refused to attend classes, Mochtar went to their dormitory (at Cikini 71) and pleaded with them to return. The very next day, at Mochtar's urging, all four nationalist leaders (Soekarno, Hatta, Mansyoer, and Dewantoro—the "empat serangkai") appeared at Cikini 71 to plead with the students to end their strike. The proud students steadfastly refused the humiliation imposed by the Japanese at the school.

It is remarkable that the Japanese renamed the school of medicine and all of its affiliated arms (pharmacy, dentistry, and the teaching hospital), as well as the Pasteur Institute at Bandung, but not the Eijkman Institute.[9] We speculate that Eijkman's historic German and Japanese links may explain that. Eijkman was Robert Koch's research fellow at the same time as famed Japanese scientist Shibasabura Kitazato, the discoverer of tetanus toxin in that laboratory. That is a great irony to be fully appreciated in later chapters.

Merdeka!

Merdeka translates literally as "free." When shouted by a nationalist, however, it practically translates as a demand for independence or, more precisely, for liberty from the colonial yoke. It is akin to the American cry "Give me liberty, or give me death!" In late 1945 the nationalists began to firmly understand that their declaration of independence of August 17 would require force of arms to survive. The defeated Japanese would go home, but the Dutch would return. Nationalism would cease being a cherished ideal and evolve into a very dangerous act of armed insurrection. "Merdeka!" became their battle cry.

The execution of Mochtar in July 1945 has no known link to his

Coming of Age

political beliefs. The Japanese would inject politics into his persecution, ridiculously accusing him of instigating a Minangkabau rebellion against Javanese dominance of the incipient republic. We do not know Mochtar's exact political sentiments, but can easily suppose Indonesian independence was a dream he shared. We know he was close to Mohammad Hatta, a fellow Minangkabau and intellectual and, just weeks after Mochtar's execution, the new vice president of the republic. Mochtar's nephew, Abu Hanifah, lived with Mochtar for a time in Batavia and went on to lead the strongly Islamic Masyumi nationalist political party and, later, the Laskar Hesbollah armed rebel faction during the 1945–49 war of independence. Mochtar's sons at medical school in Holland lived in Leiden with a confirmed nationalist leader, Nazir Pamuntjak. Mochtar very clearly was not averse to having his sons under the direct influence of potentially dangerous nationalist leaders. These facts point to Mochtar's very probable firm ideological alignment with that movement.

The Japanese occupiers, as already explained, were even more deeply suspicious of Hatta than the Dutch colonialists had been, and they tried on at least one occasion to assassinate him. They would have looked with suspicion at his associates, and eventually several of the STOVIA men among them would be arrested and tortured in connection with the Mochtar affair.

There can be little doubt that, as an intellectual with close ties not only to the STOVIA network of dangerous thinkers but also to confirmed Minangkabau nationalists like Hanifah and Hatta, Mochtar was known to the Kenpeitai, the military police of the Imperial Japanese Army, from near the beginning of the occupation in March 1942. But Mochtar also symbolized a future for Indonesia, and the Japanese accorded him positions of respect and authority in medicine. The Japanese cultivated this face of beneficence for the benefit of their nationalist leader supporters. As will be explained in later chapters, Mochtar's arrest, torture, and execution became a self-preserving necessity for the Japanese occupier. That crime was not primarily a cruelty aimed at him personally. However, once the Japanese committed to that course with Mochtar, deeply cruel and personal it certainly became. Mochtar had played a key role, years earlier, in scientific research that contributed to the downfall of Hideyo Noguchi, Japan's adored and most internationally prominent scientist. The rabidly nationalistic Kenpeitai certainly knew this and would have considered it direct evidence of Mochtar's anti-Japanese sentiments.

In the next chapter we shall examine Mochtar as a scientist. Understanding the accomplishments and stature of the man in that field is essential to grasping the weight of the crime of killing him. In his scientific confrontation with Noguchi over the causative germ of yellow fever, we see his promise and courage as a medical scientist. In his technical endeavors, Mochtar stood among the greatest medical minds of the early twentieth century. He worked with them, challenged their ideas, and in so doing advanced human medicine.

SIX

Excellence

Most accomplished scientists will attest that early in their careers someone helped them climb over the formidable obstacles to succeed and excel. Few reach scientific heights singlehandedly. Many benefit from having a series of such mentors who actively cultivate their stepwise success. Mochtar launched himself on his path to becoming an internationally known and respected scientist when he allied with a Dutch mentor in the Mandailing region of North Sumatra. As in all such relationships, the mentor chose him as a worthy investment.

The eventual acquisition of skill and confidence as a master of scientific endeavor amounts to a long and meticulously guided process down an extremely narrow lane of science. Schools of medicine, on the other hand, effectively cram vast amounts of acquired human knowledge of the art and practice into young minds. Medicine or science each requires a substantial intellect and steely determination, but mastery of science demands closer and more prolonged mentoring within a highly specialized niche of scientific progress. Put another way, the physician acquires broad knowledge and specific skills, while the scientist acquires broad skills and specific knowledge. Mochtar, as both physician and Minangkabau, would have found the chance of advancing human knowledge of medicine as a scientist enormously appealing. When it came, he seized his opportunity.

As a newly minted physician in 1916, Mochtar was obliged to serve at a location chosen by the government. All the way up until 2007, licensing as a physician in Indonesia required two years of service in the government healthcare system, regardless of where one was educated or who paid the expenses of that education, be it in Indonesia or abroad. This almost always meant being posted to a remote location lacking in voluntary doctors due to isolation, poverty, physical discomfort, and the risk of endemic infectious diseases.

The government assigned Mochtar to serve at Penyabungan, in remote northwestern Sumatra. As fate would have it, this medical posting was in the region of Mandailing, where in 1917 the famous W.A.P. Schüffner and soon to be famous N. H. Swellengrebel would conduct groundbreaking longitudinal microscopic surveys in the study of malaria epidemiology.[1]

Schüffner's work became widely cited, was reprinted in English in 1938, and is today considered a classic in modern malariology for its exquisite attention to the composition of parasite stages in blood across age groups and time.[2] The work at Mandailing may also have been the genesis of "Schüffner's dots," known today to anyone trained in the microscopic diagnosis of malaria as the bright red speckling of stained red blood cells infected by the parasite *Plasmodium vivax*.

Malariologists almost always recruit local medical talent into their field efforts, as a routine and often useful professional courtesy. It is therefore quite likely that the Dutch doctors appeared one day at the clinic in Penyabungan and politely invited Mochtar to join in the work of the research team. Schüffner's team stayed in Mandailing for most of 1917 and part of 1918. Its leader would have had ample opportunity to watch the young Dr. Mochtar work and to see the spark of scientific promise in this potential protégé.

A few years later, Mochtar was Schüffner's student at the University of Amsterdam. In his 1926 doctoral thesis Mochtar offered his thanks to Schüffner and cited the time under his direct supervision in the "Sumatran malaria paradise." He also thanked Swellengrebel for their time together in Penyabungan. A photograph shows the very young Mochtar seated next to a standing Dutch doctor, possibly Swellengrebel, in front of the research team's residence at Penyabungan.

Participating in the classical studies of malaria epidemiology conducted there, and apparently deeply impressing Schüffner, Mochtar found his chance to excel and to take a quantum leap in his professional development that was offered to a rare few. He made that leap and went far.

Leptospirosis and Yellow Fever

W.A.P. Schüffner was a prolific clinical, laboratory and field investigator. In addition to his seminal work in malaria (a parasitic infection), he broke new ground in understanding Weil's disease (a bacterial infection). This malady had been described clinically in 1886, and in 1915 Japanese scientists identified the cause, a long and distinctly corkscrew-shaped bacterium. Today we know these leptospires cause a dizzying array of clinical manifestations, affecting almost any organ system. These many varieties of the same infection had been known by as many common names such as rat-catcher's yellows, contagious jaundice, canicola fever, cane field fever, and Fort Bragg fever. Today these seemingly distinct diseases are collectively and more accurately referred to as a single disease, leptospirosis.

Clinical leptospirosis begins innocently. The flu-like symptoms of the first phase of infection graduate to any one of several severe manifestations (in some patients), including liver or kidney failure, respiratory distress, or meningitis. The causative bacteria appear in the blood only during the mild early phase, and thereafter are restricted to the affected organ system.

This changing behavior and broad range of illnesses, along with inaccessibility to the tissues they invade, makes the diagnosis of leptospirosis in ill patients very difficult. These facts largely explain the medical confusion surrounding leptospirosis in the early twentieth century.

In the 1920s, the range of diseases caused by the leptospires and the means of their transmission to humans remained largely unmapped. Some diseases were not yet recognized as being caused by leptospires, and others caused by the then still mysterious viruses were wrongly suspected as being leptospirosis. As described by Terpstra, the discovery of leptospires as the cause of Weil's disease launched vigorous efforts to demonstrate the bacterium as the cause of yellow fever—then a dreaded epidemic disease responsible for a great deal of mortality all across the Americas and Africa.[3]

Weil's disease and yellow fever indeed shared some important clinical and epidemiological features, and some scientists considered yellow fever likely to be yet another manifestation of leptospirosis. It was a reasonable and rational supposition.

Walter Reed and colleagues in Cuba had already demonstrated, two decades earlier, the fact that yellow fever was transmitted by mosquitoes rather than by person-to-person contact or from the things that people touch (fomites). Weil's disease similarly appeared not to be communicable between humans. More important, a highly distinguished and internationally famous bacteriologist, Dr. Hideyo Noguchi, published papers between 1919 and 1922 that described a species of leptospire, which he named *Leptospira icteroides*, as the likely cause of yellow fever.

Schüffner would put Mochtar to work on the leptospires in his laboratory in Amsterdam, as he did with Raden Soesilo (STOVIA fellow student and later Mochtar's colleague at the Eijkman Institute and ultimately fellow martyr) two years earlier. More specifically, Schüffner disbelieved the yellow fever–leptospire hypothesis, and so he encouraged Mochtar to put the hypothesis to very hard laboratory testing. This brought Mochtar's academic career across the immense, shining, and tragic path of Dr. Noguchi.[4]

Dr. Hideyo Noguchi

In 1905 Schaudinn and Hoffman described the bacterium *Treponema pallidum* in patients with acute syphilis. They called it "pallidum" because of the extreme difficulty of properly staining the microbe—it appeared pallid in their chemically stained preparations. This characteristic continues to vex pathologists to the present day. In 1913 the young, bright, and breathtakingly energetic Dr. Hideyo Noguchi of Japan (working at the Rockefeller Foundation in New York) proved that *Treponema pallidum* caused a dreaded neurological disease commonly occurring a decade or so after acute syphilis. Previously not firmly linked to the acute infection, doctors called the disease "general paralysis of the insane," and it was managed as a psychiatric problem. Noguchi's discovery revealed it as an infection, and it became known as tertiary syphilis or neurosyphilis.

Before the dawn of antibiotic therapies in the 1940s, syphilis rep-

resented a hugely important social, clinical, and public health problem. Much like HIV before the advent of anti-retroviral therapies,
syphilis carried a sentence of severe social ostracism and, very often,
a slow and agonizing death. The late-stage bacterium invades the
brain, where Noguchi found it by exhaustive microscopic searches
of stained tissue sections collected at autopsy. Patients with late-
stage syphilis were confined to asylums to await the onset of insanity and death, almost invariably within three or four years of onset
and usually a decade or more after acquiring the primary infection.

Noguchi's discovery was a critical step in the direction of a cure
for neurosyphilis. In the last ten years of Noguchi's abbreviated life,
he would be nominated for the Nobel Prize eight times. The emperor
of Japan heaped honors upon him, as did many nations, including
France, which bestowed the Legion of Merit on Noguchi. When he
traveled to foreign capitals, his picture appeared in local newspapers.
Ecuador commissioned him as a colonel in their army. Noguchi's
heroic stature in the public eye for leading progress against such a
dreaded and widespread disease placed him in the company of such
giants as Koch and Pasteur.

When the Austrian psychiatrist Wagner-Jauregg discovered that the
fevers of malaria permanently cured neurosyphilis in some patients,
he won the 1927 Nobel Prize for Medicine. His innovative treatment,
however, was poorly efficacious and quite dangerous—only a third of
patients recovered their health, and about one in ten did not survive
the intense malaria fevers required for therapeutic success against
neurosyphilis. Modern treatment of syphilis with penicillin is virtually 100 percent effective and brings harm to almost no one. Had
Noguchi survived to the dawn of such therapies, just over the horizon, he would perhaps have also been awarded the Nobel Prize for
his original discovery of a bacterial cause of general paralysis of the
insane. That prize is not awarded posthumously.

Noguchi's expertise reached across a broad range of the burgeon-
ing field of microbiology. His publications begin in 1902 and end
in 1929, a year after his death. In that span he published an astonishing 116 scientific papers. All of these are in English, a language
he taught himself as a young man. Noguchi also completely over-
came the daunting obstacles of being born into grinding poverty and

of losing the use of one of his hands to a severe burn injury as an infant. Noguchi faced several compelling reasons to fail in medicine and science, and each one he brushed aside as mere inconveniences.

His American journey began when he showed up on the laboratory doorstep of Simon Flexner at University of Pennsylvania in Philadelphia, penniless and jobless. Flexner, immortalized in the name of an important intestinal germ, *Shigella flexneri*, would become a second father to Noguchi. He took Noguchi in, trained him, and nurtured his progress all the way up to his premature death. Noguchi began his scientific career with seven years of elegant laboratory studies on snake venoms. This journeyman work equipped him with powerful serological techniques and skills he would later harness in his pursuits on a wide array of human infections.

In 1909 he began contributing work on syphilis and on complement fixation techniques for its diagnosis. He moved on to the leptospires (the genus *Leptospira*, which he described and named). His published work on these organisms and on yellow fever begins in 1919 and ceases in 1922. He then moved on to Rocky Mountain spotted fever (a dreaded tick-borne infection known to North Americans), leishmaniasis (a parasitic infection common in Central and South America), and a series of seminal papers on Oroyo fever (bartonellosis of the Andes region) dominate his last pieces of work.

In 1919, Noguchi published reports in highly prestigious journals of medicine and science (*Proceedings of the National Academy of Sciences* and the *Journal of Experimental Medicine*) that linked a particular species (or serotype) of leptospire to yellow fever. He wrote in one of these, "Fortunately, I was successful in detecting in certain cases of yellow fever by culture methods and by guinea pig inoculation a particular spiral organism which I have since named *Leptospira icteroides.*"[5] He closed his report with an appropriately cautious note: "Its standing as the inciting agent of yellow fever will have to be regarded as not yet certainly established."

When a scientist publishes a finding in a prestigious journal of science, he or she is saying, in effect, "This is an important discovery." The editors and peers who critically examine that claim must tend to agree, both technically and with regard to overall importance. The 1919 papers by Noguchi heralded a potentially enormous advance in medicine: the cause (and therefore, later, cure) of yellow fever in humans. Noguchi would have to deal with the "not yet certainly established" verbiage to truly bag this historic trophy.

The challenge of nailing down this cause-and-effect hypothesis was formidable. Noguchi was dealing with microorganisms that were ubiquitous, hugely diverse, difficult to isolate and culture, and nearly impossible to classify taxonomically. That task in that age may be compared to a detective seeking a criminal on the basis of a physical description limited to "ordinary-looking fellow." Noguchi courageously trod upon technically treacherous ground. Ultimately he stumbled.

Unlike many important bacterial pathogens, the varieties of leptospires cannot be distinguished under the microscope or in test tube cultures. By the diagnostic standards of the time they appeared to all be the same microbe. Noguchi set out to demonstrate they were different and thereby explain the wide array of seemingly distinct diseases caused by them. He used animals induced to have immune responses that protected against some leptospire isolates but not against others. He reasoned these were antigenically distinct and therefore taxonomically distinct, that is, separate species. In other words, he allowed antibody responses in his lab animals to detect differences at the molecular level that no microscope or culture tube could see. It was technically brilliant work. The detective began to learn how to sort "ordinary-looking fellows" to find his criminal.

Noguchi collected cultures of leptospires isolated from patients with Weil's disease (*Leptospira ictohaemorrhagiae*) and from patients with yellow fever isolated at Guayaquil, Ecuador (*Leptospira icteroides*). He demonstrated that animals inoculated with isolates from each of these allegedly distinct species were protected against further inoculations of that species. When animals with immunity against *L. icteroides* were challenged with *L. ictohaemorrhagiae*, they appeared to be immune, albeit imperfectly. Thus the spirochetes known to cause Weil's disease appeared to be the same as those taken from patients with yellow fever. However, Noguchi later used a finer test of a reaction called the Pfeiffer phenomenon to draw the conclusion that the two groups were closely related but distinct. Later, he would be successfully challenged on this very refined technical point.

In the meantime, Noguchi took his findings with *L. icteroides* into the tricky domains of epidemiology and public health. The vagaries of unrecognized confusion (in the choosing, observing, or treatment of groups being compared) in those fields served to cement his conviction of cause and effect. The field evidence badly misled him.

Noguchi prepared a vaccine against *L. icteroides* and injected it into 427 people in Peru. This cohort experienced only 5 cases of yellow fever, whereas the unvaccinated general population (its total number, remarkably, not specified) experienced 386 cases (217 of them fatal) in the same period. He did not consider the denominators of risk estimation (we don't know what they were), and convinced himself (and many others) that there had been vaccine-induced protection. However, if the general population numbered 33,000, for example, there would be no protective effect. Further, had the outbreak not reached those vaccinated (because of geographic separation, for example), the evidence of protection would also crumble. Noguchi did not seem to recognize these analytical hazards.

In the wake of this flawed work, and because of Noguchi's huge influence with Simon Flexner (founding director of the Rockefeller), the Foundation prepared 20,000 doses of the *L. icteroides* vaccine and administered it in uncontrolled trials in Ecuador, Brazil, Mexico, and Peru. They did the vaccinations, unwisely, in conjunction with anti-mosquito measures. The number of cases of yellow fever in trial areas fell precipitously. Noguchi's vaccine was presumed to have played a defining role. The impact of the anti-mosquito measures, even then known as an effective device against yellow fever, was somehow discounted. By 1925, Noguchi and his patrons earnestly believed he had discovered the cause of yellow fever and had invented a vaccine for its prevention.

In 1926, Noguchi's seemingly firm evidence that *L. icteroides* caused yellow fever faced its first challenge in the form of contradictory laboratory evidence. Max Theiler and Andrew Sellards at Harvard published a devastating cross-examination of Noguchi's Pfeiffer phenomenon data on *L. icteroides* (yellow fever) and *L. ictohaemorrhagiae* (Weil's disease).[6] They deemed the two species to be identical, closing their paper with an exceedingly polite but direct assault upon Noguchi's hypothesis: "One is confronted with possibilities too radical for detailed discussion at present, the extremes being that Weil's disease and yellow fever may be etiologically identical, or that the leptospira may have no etiological relationship to yellow fever." To a scientist like Noguchi who had staked his formidable reputation on the link between leptospires and yellow fever, Theiler and Sellards had thrown down a very serious challenge. It would have been clear to those in the field that Weil's disease and yellow fever were certainly not caused by the same microbe. What Theiler and Sellards were saying was very clear—the leptospira appear to have nothing to do with yellow fever. Mochtar would weigh in shortly thereafter with a decisive blow.

In his 1926 doctoral dissertation, Achmad Mochtar, then an obscure scientist from the Netherlands East Indies, challenged Noguchi's hypothesis. Working at the busy leptospirosis laboratory of W.A.P. Schüffner in Amsterdam, he directly examined the possible relationship between *L. icteroides* and yellow fever. Mochtar's findings devastated Noguchi's hypothetical link and very probably unwittingly provided his future Japanese captors with motivation for even greater persecution.

In his published 1927 review of Mochtar's thesis, B. M. van Driel wrote, "The research of Mochtar is very important for appraisal of the question if *Leptospira icteroides* actually causes yellow fever or not."[7] Using a more refined and precise technique than that of Theiler and Sellards, Mochtar also declared *L. ictohaemorrhagiae* and *L. icteroides* to be the same organism. This meant the leptospires taken from yellow fever patients were almost certainly not the cause of that illness. He concluded that Noguchi's *L. icteroides* isolated from patients with yellow fever were very likely taken from patients simultaneously infected with both yellow fever and Weil's disease.

Mochtar carried his assault on Noguchi's hypothesis even farther. He demonstrated that mosquitoes could not transmit *L. icteroides*, and dismissed Noguchi's positive findings as simply mechanical transmission on mosquito mouthparts. When a germ simply contaminates an insect's mouthparts, it is vastly less efficient (and insignificant in a public health sense) than invading and multiplying within that insect, which the cause of yellow fever, whatever it happened to be, was supposed to do.

This was a critical point: the link between mosquitoes and yellow fever, thanks to Walter Reed, was firm. Any hypothesis putting forth a causative microbe had to be reconciled with this fact. The germ needed to be harbored and amplified by mosquitoes, not simply surviving for a few minutes on their feeding parts. Today we know the virus responsible for yellow fever indeed invades mosquito tissues and vastly expands its numbers therein.

The Downfall of Noguchi's Hypothesis and His Death

In 1926 the West African Yellow Fever Commission of the Rockefeller Foundation had assigned Dr. Henry Beeuwkes to Lagos, Nigeria. His boss, Dr. Fredrick Russell (director of the famous International Health Division of that foundation), sent him to conduct experiments designed to prove that *L. icteroides* caused African yellow fever, then viewed as proven for American yellow fever. Beeuwkes reported contrary findings from Africa. He could not find evidence of the leptospire being linked to yellow fever in people or mosquitoes. In April 1927 Russell received a telegram from Beeuwkes in Amsterdam. He had been visiting Schüffner's laboratory and conveyed the finding (Mochtar's just-published thesis) that *L. icteroides* and *L. ictohaemorrhagiae* were serologically indistinct.[8] Credible evidence was mounting that Noguchi had committed a monumental error.

In August 1927 a besieged Noguchi retreated to his cabin in the New York woods. According to Isabel Plesset, he carried with him the "Schüffner papers" to study.[9] This was almost certainly Mochtar's newly published thesis.

Ironically, Noguchi's colleagues at the Rockefeller Foundation published the definitive final assault on his hypothesis in early 1928. Adrian Stokes, J. H. Bauer, and N. Paul Hudson published a landmark paper innocently titled "The Transmission of Yellow Fever to Macacus rhesus" in the *Journal of the American Medical Association*. Their work constituted the first application of Koch's postulates (a description of the evidence necessary to link a microbe to a particular disease) to demonstrate a virus as the cause of a human disease. This paper is widely cited as the first evidence for a virus being the cause of yellow fever, although the authors did not isolate the virus. They simply proved that the causative germ passed through filters capable of netting all known bacteria.[10] Earlier work on tobacco mosaic virus (a disease of plants) pointed to nonfilterable germs being the then largely mysterious viruses.

The work by Stokes and colleagues was conducted at the Rockefeller Foundation laboratory at Accra, Ghana (then called the Gold Coast). They imported macaques from Asia as the animal model in order to rule out the possibility of extant or prior infections of the experimental monkeys with yellow fever (which does not occur in Asia). The animals were kept in mosquito-proofed cages to prevent natural exposure. As the work neared completion, Stokes accidentally acquired the infection in his laboratory and died of yellow fever.

With Stokes freshly in his grave, Noguchi's ardent supporters at the Rockefeller arranged for Noguchi to travel to Africa to reconcile the new data to his hypothesis. In the background, Simon Flexner pushed to somehow vindicate Noguchi. Flexner, too, had already committed himself scientifically to Noguchi's *L. icteroides* causing yellow fever. The mission at this point was to prove that American and African yellow fever were different disease entities: leptospiral in the Americas and viral in Africa. That outcome would salvage both Noguchi's and Flexner's reputations, among others. It is unclear, however, what technical strategy Noguchi (or Flexner) actually had in mind. The work he conducted there was never published.

On October 22, 1927, a sullen Noguchi set sail for Africa, asking that no one see him off.[11] Noguchi arrived at Accra and set about his usual frenetic pace of work. Flexner had given explicit orders that Noguchi was to be denied nothing in his work. Other scientists at Accra and Lagos quickly began to complain to New York that Noguchi was consuming vast resources and crippling their own work. By spring of 1928, Noguchi had used more than four hundred monkeys in his experiments, and yet he had reported nothing back to New York.

Early in that same year, Sawyer replaced Russell as leader of the powerful international section of the Rockefeller. Sawyer had far less patience for and confidence in Noguchi. Rather than wait for Noguchi to work through the problem, he demanded his own quick solution to the question of the cause of American yellow fever. He arranged for the shipment to Accra of six sera from survivors of the yellow fever epidemic at Rio de Janeiro in Brazil in early 1928. Sawyer instructed that the sera be transferred into monkeys injected with sera from West African acute yellow fever patients. If those monkeys were protected from onset of yellow fever, Sawyer reasoned, it meant African and American yellow fever had a shared cause. The Brazilian sera protected the monkeys at Accra exposed to local yellow fever. Noguchi's last hope at redemption vanished with that simple experiment. American and African yellow fever had a shared cause, and it was not leptospiral. Noguchi surely was aware of these findings out of the same laboratory where he worked.

The pressure on Noguchi to reconcile *L. icteroides* with yellow fever must have been crushing. A report published in *Time* magazine on the very day of Noguchi's death, May 21, 1928, gives some idea:

> Yellow fever has been stamped out in the Americas; it still rages on the coast of West Africa. Noguchi discovered that American yellow fever was caused by a tiny organism which he named *Leptospira icteroides*: was carried by a common lady mosquito, *Stegomyia calopus*; that guinea pigs could be infected with the organism; that mosquito could carry the infection from one animal to another; that a horse serum could be prepared that could cure the disease if administered shortly after the infection. These facts are known, the disease was conquered. The same process must be applied to West Africa. For over two years a Commission of the Rockefeller Foundation has been at work on the problem in the U.S. and Africa. Progress has been held up because none of the experimental animals would contract the African form of yellow fever. In the end it was Dr. Noguchi himself who went to Accra on the west coast of Africa to experiment, was there taken to the hospital with yellow fever. On the fifth day when his high temperature was reluctantly dropping and the second stage of the disease had set in, he had a monkey from India (*Macacus rhesus*) inoculated with infected blood. The monkey died twelve days later from a severe case of yellow fever. Fifty more monkeys were inoculated and succumbed. Finally serum from the blood of patient Noguchi, recovering from the yellow fever, was administered and the protective antibodies prevented animals from contracting yellow fever from a subsequent injection of the germ. Bacteriologist Noguchi by his experiment has found the invading West African organ-

ism to a more vicious member of the American leptospire family, is now working on a vaccine.

The author of the report is not identified. Whoever it was, he or she was apparently in communication with people close to the work in Accra. Nonetheless, there was no mention of the decisive experiment demonstrating protection against Africa yellow fever with American immune plasma. The stubborn insistence upon *L. icteroides* in the *Time* article surely reflects the strength of the lay view on this, rather than a view to be attributed to Noguchi at that very late hour.

No matter how Noguchi acquired his lethal case of yellow fever at Accra, he surely understood before becoming ill that he was wrong about *L. icteroides* and yellow fever. Some speculate that in a fit of scientific vanity, Noguchi had injected himself with the sera from yellow fever patients filtered to remove bacteria (hoping to prove his hypothesis by remaining healthy). This speculation is not supported by any known facts, and it is grossly unfair to Noguchi. He was a good enough scientist to read the data and understand that he had been wrong. He would not have killed himself in the vain hope of good data being wrong just because he wished it be so.

Regardless of method or intent, Noguchi martyred himself in the earnest pursuit of the truth and justifiably earned the admiration of the people close to him and around the world. Flexner published a touching obituary of Noguchi in *Science* magazine. In closing he gives a brief description of the extraordinary esteem his fellow Japanese citizens held for Noguchi before and especially after his death. The emperor of Japan, who had decorated Noguchi in 1915, did so again posthumously with one of the highest classes of the Order of the Rising Sun with gold and silver stars. His birthplace was immediately acquired after his death and turned into a shrine. Flexner writes, "The spirit of science will surely hover over this shrine, and in accordance with the genius of his countrymen, it will attract worshipers to whom the name Hideyo Noguchi will be a sacred emblem of love of his fellow man."[12]

As early as 1937 the Hideyo Noguchi Foundation operated an office in Tokyo. The extraordinary popular admiration for the stellar scientist remains undiminished. In 1979 the Japanese government funded the creation of the Noguchi Memorial Institute for Medical Research at Legon, just outside of Accra, Ghana. The institute's first director was Dr. Francis Nkrumah, son of the famous founder of the nation of Ghana and the African unity movement. Since 2004, Noguchi's portrait has appeared on the 1,000 yen note of Japan. Finally, the government of Japan in 2006 established the Noguchi Prize for Medicine in Africa, carrying an extraordinary 100 million yen prize. Noguchi was in his time, and remains today, a precious gem of Japanese intellectual pride.

The name and reputation of Hideyo Noguchi likely played a role in what befell Achmad Mochtar, through the misguided and inflamed nationalistic pride of his captors. Noguchi and the venerated memory of his astonishing humanism, commitment, and accomplishments did not. The honors bestowed upon this bright light of the early twentieth century should not in any way be diminished by the conduct of countrymen whom Noguchi himself would surely have considered both repugnant and an affront to everything his endeavors and life stood for. As his many accomplishments decisively demonstrate, Hideyo Noguchi served all of humanity rather than just his adoring native nation.

Science with Feeling

Mochtar arrived in Amsterdam in 1920, apparently having no experience or knowledge of the leptospires. Schüffner immediately put him into the harness of academic rigor within this very specific niche. At least one source suggests that Schüffner had both a personal dislike of Noguchi and serious doubts about *L. icteroides*. Another author, J. F. Schacher, reviewing Plesset's book *Noguchi and His Patrons*, recalled his mentor in 1952 complaining that Noguchi made three mistakes: "one was being too 'cocksure' that spirochete was the cause of yellow fever, the second was in not seeing that he was wrong, and the third was in allowing people who were hated even more than he was to champion the cause."[13] Schacher's mentor here refers to the controversial Simon Flexner as champion.

Science can often be driven by force or clash of personalities. If a scientist takes a personal dislike of another scientist, he will often seize an opportunity to aim the weapon of science at the work and reputation of the scientist whom he disfavors. Provided the rules of rigorous science remain intact, this personal pettiness can be tolerated and is often even considered healthy in the intercourse of science. Schüffner may well have put Noguchi's *L. icteroides* in his proverbial scientific crosshairs because he did not like the man. If so, the gun he took aim with was Achmad Mochtar.

A contemporary reading of an English translation of Mochtar's thesis (it was published in Dutch) indeed appears provocative. As has been explained, Mochtar confronted Noguchi's hypothesis head-on across several fronts. He dared venture explanations of Noguchi's findings in both yellow fever patients and mosquitoes as essentially the imperfect practice of science. Mochtar closed his dissertation with conclusion no. 6: "The etiology of the yellow fever remains unknown despite the findings of Noguchi."[14]

One cannot help but see the editorial hand of Schüffner in this bold and ultimately unnecessary overt hostility. The sentence could have ended with "unknown," without the finger pointing. In the culture of science, this amounted to a face slap, and it was exceptionally direct language from a freshly minted PhD toward a towering figure of science and medicine. However, Mochtar had the proxy of Schüffner, who could rightfully consider himself Noguchi's peer. The expressed hostility supports the supposition that Schüffner had an axe to grind with Noguchi. It would surely have struck the nerve of Japanese nationalists, especially after Noguchi's martyrdom. According to his nephew Abu Hanifah, when the Kenpeitai searched Mochtar's residence in October 1944, they carried away only one item—a copy of his 1926 doctoral dissertation.[15]

This exemplifies the struggle among scientists to distinguish between what is thought and what is real. Noguchi thought *L. icteroides* caused yellow fever. He strove hard to link that to reality. Mochtar and others, as is the right and duty of scientists, nullified that linkage for the simple reason that it was, in fact, imagined.

The possible link between this kind of fair scientific combat— Mochtar and Schüffner played within the rules of science, despite any personal feelings—and the subsequent persecution of Achmad Mochtar by the Japanese Kenpeitai will be discussed later. In the current context, one can see in this Noguchi–yellow fever episode both Mochtar's scientific courage and his technical excellence. This young, unheralded doctor from Sumatra successfully challenged one the greatest and most famous minds in medicine of the early twentieth century.

No documentation of Mochtar's thoughts on Noguchi and his death is known. He appears to have simply carried on with his work on the leptospires of Netherlands East Indies (where yellow fever does not occur). A good scientist does not gloat at victory over another. That is very bad form, and there is no record of it from either Mochtar or Schüffner. It seems very likely that Mochtar, the good scientist, would have rarely thought of poor Noguchi until the Kenpeitai put his own thesis in front of him in their Jakarta prison in 1944.

Investigator Mochtar

In 1926 Mochtar shared with Max Theiler the distinction of offering a technically sound challenge to Noguchi's then widely accepted hypothesis. Theiler would go on to study the virus of yellow fever, develop a means of cultivating it, and, in so doing, create an effective vaccine against it. He would win the Nobel Prize for Medicine in 1951 for this work.

In 1927, Mochtar's first post-thesis publication likely represents a full description of the serological technology he and Schüffner (and other students) developed in the study of leptospires. This work represents one of the foundations of the technological means of characterizing the many "tribes" of leptospires occurring in Nature. The technique involved microscopically observing the agglutination (clumping together) of leptospira grown in culture when mixed with plasma containing antibodies against specific groups of leptospires. Recall that Noguchi and Theiler each used the course of disease in inoculated animals to understand relationships among leptospires. The methods of Schüffner and Mochtar opened the door to far more precise and efficient laboratory testing. In effect, they removed the test animals and all of their maintenance and physiological vagaries from the analysis. They let the antibodies speak directly to tribe identity by spotting differences at the molecular level. This technology remains the gold standard for the serological classification of the leptospires today.

When Mochtar returned to Indonesia, he took up residence at Bengkulu on the southwestern coast of Sumatra. In 1929 he published a report of the parasitic worm that causes filariasis (and, in chronic stages, disfiguring elephantiasis) in that region. His later published papers, almost all of them on serological testing of leptospire isolates, came from a government laboratory at Semarang, on the northern coast of central Java. He spent several years in Semarang. In 1934 he published a paper in conjunction with R. M. Djoehana and M. Sardjito, both of the Eijkman Institute. Finally, in 1937, his name appears in the roster of scientific staff at Eijkman. He was at last part of the era's greatest institute for tropical medicine and entering a prolific period as a scientist.

At Eijkman Mochtar assumed broader bacteriological responsibilities. He was still publishing prolifically in leptospirosis with Dutch colleagues H. Esseveld and W. A. Collier and with Indonesian colleague M. Sardjito, but he also published two papers on cholera with W. K. Mertens and J. K. Baars, both in 1938, and another in 1939 (his most prolific year, with nine papers).

In 1940 Mochtar published on a fluorescent diagnostic test for tuberculosis. In the same year he published five other papers, alone and with colleagues Bahder Djohan and W. A. Collier, on leptospirosis. His last prolific year was 1941, with six publications. In these he continued his dedication to leptospirosis, along with broadening interests in internal medicine and chemistry. His 1941 publications included collaborations with Dutch (A. G. van Veen, C. A. de Reede, and D. Rikebusch) and Indonesian (Wahab and B. Djohan) co-workers.

Mochtar's last known publication appeared in January 1943. It listed December 1942 as the date it was received and accepted. It was written in German and published in the *Japanese Journal of Veterinary Medicine*. The abstract was presented in Japanese kanji.

Dr. Achmad Mochtar, up to the invasion of his homeland by the Imperial Japanese Army, contributed enduringly significant work in the field of leptospirosis. He and his mentor, W.A.P. Schüffner, deserve credit for pioneering the means of classifying leptospire bacteria that remains the gold standard in clinical and research diagnostics up to the present day, though of course now using improved modern biotechnology.

Achmad Mochtar had indeed come very far from Bonjol, West Sumatra. He not only gathered the wisdom of the outside world, as demanded by Minangkabau tradition, but he also had informed and increased it. The coming fulfillment of an obscure Javanese prophecy, the hope-inspiring, postcolonial vision of Joyoboyo, would see Mochtar's life, dedication, and accomplishments all turned horribly inside out. That topsy-turvy new world was managed by people driven to demonstrate lies as truth—the antithesis of Mochtar's intellectual being. His courage, intellectual honesty, hard work, and cultivated intellect in that twisted new world of wartime occupation would ultimately be his undoing.

SEVEN

New Reality

Shame

During an interview in 2010, Dr. Asikin Hanafiah, Mochtar's nephew, recalled the day in early March 1942 when the Japanese army poured into Batavia on foot, bicycles, commandeered sedans, and ordinary trucks. He was nine years old. On an otherwise nearly abandoned and quiet city street, Asikin saw a group of Dutch soldiers sitting and smoking cigarettes leisurely atop their mighty armored vehicle bristling with menacing weapons. They seemed bored and waiting for something. In a moment they all craned their heads to look in the same direction. Asikin followed their gaze to see a lone Japanese trooper, rifle slung over his shoulder, pedal slowly around a street corner on a rickety old bicycle. The Japanese trooper, seeing his enemy, stopped and stood astride his bicycle. The Dutch soldiers did not move at first, but then in near unison, they raised their hands in surrender. The Japanese soldier approached almost curiously and motioned for them to dismount the vehicle. He disarmed them, cast their cold weapons into a pile next to the idle war wagon, and marched them off—his rifle still slung on his back as he pushed the bike behind the column of docile prisoners.

Even sixty-eight years later Asikin described, with gleaming wonderment, how he stood dumbstruck with mouth agape, both at the event and the profound, almost palpable transformation he immediately sensed in his psyche. A supposition of the innate superiority of the white rulers of the East Indies, though unspoken and certainly not taught at home, had nonetheless crept into his young consciousness. The faintly comic scene he witnessed washed away for all time (Asikin declared firmly) the corollary of that supposition—an innate sense of racial inferiority. It had been, he then realized, like an ugly stain he had no longer noticed. Once vanished, its prior presence seemed obvious and shameful. An intense utter joy and pride at its sudden absence welled up powerfully in his heart. And, at the time, he directed his enormous gratitude to the Japanese invaders for that astonishing cleansing.

Similar scenes and emotions occurred all across the East Indies. The Dutch colonial forces, the KNIL, were more like a police force than an army. Their strategy, tactics, and utility had been inward looking, typically dealing with poorly armed insurgents, rebellious spasms, or internecine conflicts within their fractious territories. These issues certainly had occupied them fully for several hundred years. An invading foreign army breaching the outer defenses of Indochina, Burma, Malaya, and the Philippines had not been considered even remotely possible. The KNIL effectively accepted defeat the moment the Japanese put boots on Java. They were not even slightly prepared to deal with mortal combat against a formidable and fiercely determined invading army, even one on stolen bicycles.

The cost of such negligence would be very steep. Among the several hundred thousand Dutch interred on Java and elsewhere, all would suffer tremendously, and many thousands would not survive the war in a harsh captivity. More Dutch would perish after the war when their army returned to reclaim the colony. All of this suffering and loss, however, shrinks to triviality compared with the misery and lives lost among Indonesians during and after the Japanese occupation. The fatal arrogance of the colonizers of East Asia (Dutch, British, French, Portuguese, and American) permitted the cataclysm of Japan's aggression and military success all across the region. Haughty colonial paternalism for Asians had utterly failed them.

The already morally shaky foundations of colonialism as an institution had been irreversibly shattered—not by Imperial Japan's sweeping victories but by the inability of the colonialists to stop them. The brutish occupier would extract a horrific price from the colonized for the bumptious neglect of the colonizers. Europeans and Americans had fled en masse as the Japanese forces descended upon their colonies, leaving the colonized masses to fend for themselves with this cruel new master. The enterprise of colonial rule in Asia had been revealed for what it was—shameful. The scene witnessed by the boy Asikin, the emotions it inspired in him, and the sheer terror of the wholesale massacres that followed firmly dictated that colonial imperialism was forever finished in the Asian sphere.

Indonesia, like its neighbors, would have to endure a final colonial occupation by the Japanese imperialists. They could not know of the Allied victory to come. Indeed in April 1942, that appeared highly implausible. But the Indonesians had *Pralembang Joyoboyo* and acted in anticipation of a quick exit by this harsh new master. At the time they could not imagine how or when the Japanese would leave—they seemed to be settling in for permanence. The nationalist leaders dealing with that new resident master required all of the political savvy, endurance, resolve, and survival instincts they could muster. It also invited a very dangerous and real risk in doing so: being perceived as mere instruments of a new colonial master by their political base of 70 million fellow Indonesians yearning for genuine liberty.

Tightrope

The Japanese occupiers on Java quickly understood that indigenous political currents required their attention and delicate management. With Dutch sovereignty abolished, the Japanese simply imposed martial law. They expediently left in the hands of capable Indonesian managers and technicians large pieces of administrative and technical infrastructure installed and perfected by the Dutch. Nonetheless the Japanese positioned themselves in absolute authority of these enterprises in order to freely obtain the commodities of Indonesia and to exert control over the nationalist factions vying for political dominance in the occupied East Indies. They also used this power to identify threats—real, imagined, or conjured—and eliminate them. Mochtar serving as vice rector under a Japanese rector of the school of medicine in Jakarta—a nest of the intelligentsia and dangerous political thinkers—exemplifies this sort of control.

The Japanese, in the first flush of victory in the East Indies, imported and installed Japanese civilian intellectuals in positions of leadership among the many civil vacancies created by the internment of the Dutch. These people were by most accounts reasoned, pragmatic, and cooperative in their new roles. Those Japanese appeared to be genuinely sympathetic with real Indonesian independence, as if they too believed the propaganda of their own military men. However, as the war turned against them, the Japanese systematically replaced them with military men. As the militarists had done in their own nation, they eventually harnessed the East Indies into a wholly military enterprise serving solely their own interests.

Playing on the nationalist slogan of freedom and independence, "Indonesia Raya" (Great Indonesia), the Japanese in Indonesia marketed their prosperity propaganda for all of Asia as "Asia Raya." They left little doubt regarding Japan's role in that new order, however. In 1942 they launched their first major propaganda campaign called "Tiga A" or "The Three A's," which were "Japan the Leader of Asia, Japan the Light of Asia, and Japan the Protector of Asia." Events soon after the Japanese defeat reveal how this propaganda could never be reconciled with actual Japanese behavior in Indonesia. Many Japanese soldiers en route to Jakarta for repatriation were waylaid and murdered by mobs of Indonesians. Abu Hanifah encountered one vigilante who had tortured and killed three Japanese troopers in West Java. The young man angrily rebuffed Hanifah's plea to show some mercy by killing them outright rather than torturing them first. "Don't you understand they were cheating us all the time? . . . May God send them directly to hell where they really belong. They did us an injustice and soiled our honor. That is why we tortured them and I am not going to be sorry about it."[1]

These mobs also took vengeance against some Indonesians perceived as too friendly to the Japanese. Hanifah shielded a Mr. Sjamsuddin in his home from murder by armed guerrillas (led by his own nephew, Chairul Saleh). The rebels explained they wanted to kill Sjamsuddin because he had served as chairman of the Three A's organization.[2] These postwar examples serve to illustrate how the touted high principles of the Japanese occupation actually played out in the eyes of the Indonesians who endured it. To the majority of Indonesians at war's end, the Japanese soldiers had richly earned the widespread spontaneous vengeance taken against them. The real behavior of the Japanese, as opposed to that of the marketed "liberator," constantly threatened the credibility of the collaborating nationalist leadership.

At the dawn of occupation the Japanese indeed had decisively shattered the Dutch colonial yoke borne by Indonesians and seemed to be that "liberator." They set about exploiting the value of that rational impression. The Japanese created a political system for the East Indies symbolized by what they represented as the *empat serangkai*, or four-leafed clover. Each leaf represented one of the four strongest Indonesian nationalist leaders, each supported by the essential Japanese stem. The occupiers recognized the four domineering leaders and the ideological or ethnic factions they represented: Islamic, Kiai Hadji Mas Mansyoer; Javanese royalist, Ki Hadjar Dewantoro; Sumatran secular nationalist, Mohammad Hatta; and Javanese secular nationalist, Soekarno. Cadres of committed nationalists, from the elite to ordinary workers, possessed loyalties to one of these leaders. The empat serangkai embodied the nationalist hopes and dreams of Indonesians, and their followers trusted those men to realize that vision.

The Japanese stem demanded loyalty to it by those men, a leaf without a stem being doomed. The occupier thus mitigated risk of rebellion by seeming to empower the nationalists while not actually surrendering the political destiny of the East Indies to Indonesians. Up to the moment of their surrender, the Japanese firmly held the reins of government, yielding no real authority to any of the nationalist leaders. The nationalists had to await victory by Japan in their Pacific War.

All of the empat serangkai leaders, excepting Soekarno, would later each plead directly to the senior-most Japanese military authorities (to whom they had access and influence, but not a shred of authority) to spare the life of Achmad Mochtar.[3] On each occasion those officers expressed sympathy but sheepishly complained of their lack of authority over the Kenpeitai (to whom the empat serangkai had no access). The improbability of sincerity in this explanation from the Japanese occupation leaders bears more discussion later.

The empat serangkai had to walk a very fine line with the Japanese occupation government. Their solid anti-Dutch, nationalist credentials stood them in good stead with the Japanese: "the enemy of my enemy is my friend." While they enjoyed a broad base of nationalist political support from their fellow Indonesians, it was by no means beyond challenge or threat. Japanese hands on the reins of government, if prolonged any more than necessary, would certainly undermine that base. So too would cruelty directed at Indonesians engaged in enterprises endorsed and supported by the nationalist leaders, like the romusha labor program.

The heavily armed Japanese "liberator" certainly had all the earmarks of a new colonial master. They could easily and disastrously turn that enemy-of-my-enemy axiom on its head for the Indonesian masses: "the friend of my enemy is my enemy." Seventy million Indonesians might come to view their nationalist leadership in that light—friends with their enemy, a new colonizer. The eyes and ears of the Indonesian masses were acutely focused and tuned to the words and actions of the empat serangkai in their dealings with this new foreign master. Open rebellion could be the consequence of a simple misstep or miscalculation by any segment of the clover, especially its stem.

The Japanese understood this delicacy and worked to mitigate it for their Indonesian nationalist friends. They elevated and honored them—Soekarno and Hatta were decorated for their efforts on behalf of the empire in November 1943 in Tokyo by Emperor Hirohito himself—and even permitted open aspiration to nationhood. However, within the Japanese camp itself, the commitment to Indonesian nationhood was deeply insincere. Realization of this as a ploy, as expressed by Hanifah's torturing vigilante, would emerge to certainty by war's end.

The Japanese, of course, never expressed their real intentions during the occupation, but within the intimacy of their own circles they openly plotted to own most of the archipelago with victory at war's end. The vision of Indonesia Raya for the nationalists and their largely civilian Japanese sympathizers could be damned. According to Friend, "The army wanted to keep at least Sumatra after victory, and the navy all of its [Indonesia's] outer islands."[4] The Japanese acted deliberately in sparsely populated Borneo to rid it of Indonesian influence with the vision of future permanent resettlement by

Japanese citizens. Guidance provided by the Japanese Ministry of the Navy on March 14, 1942, to its forces affirms that early strategic posture. According to sources cited by Gin, it expressed, "The occupation of areas where the Navy shall act as principle administrative authority shall be directed toward their permanent retention under Japanese control. To this end, administrative and other policies shall be devised as to facilitate the organic integration of the entire region into the Japanese Empire."[5] The "Indonesia" promised by Japan, if ever delivered at all, would likely have been carved down to Java surrounded by Japanese possessions.

Japan became earnest about real Indonesian independence (per Boedi Oetomo and the Youth Pledge) only when it became obvious that the vengeful and resourceful Americans were likely to crush their vision of empire. Prime Minister Koiso formally announced plans for Indonesian independence only in September 1944. At that juncture clear-thinking Japanese leaders could see the most probable outcome of their war for Asian domination. A month earlier, the Americans had taken possession of Tinian in the Mariana Islands—putting the formidable and lethal payload of the long-range heavy bomber, the B-29 Superfortress, within reach of all major Japanese cities. Those aerial bombings immediately commenced and did not cease until August 1945. MacArthur's assault on the Philippines would begin the following month. Allied military might, decisively demonstrated by the successful penetration of Hitler's Fortress Europe in June of that year, bode very poorly for Imperial Japan. A peace treaty leaving an intact Japan began to appear as the best the Japanese could have hoped for in late 1944. Barring some military miracle, a postwar presence anywhere in Southeast Asia was already privately acknowledged as not even remotely probable.

Contingencies

Among the empat serangkai, the uncontested leader was Soekarno, widely accepted among the dominant Javanese masses as Joyoboyo's Just King in the flesh. He commanded the largest and most passionate following, and this earned him a dominating leadership position within the nationalist camp. It also earned his every utterance very close watch by the Japanese.

The tightrope Soekarno walked may be illustrated by an Indonesian newspaper article from September 1942, almost certainly published with Japanese consent, explaining to his followers the logic of how advocating noncooperation with the Dutch was not a hypocritical about-face to advocating cooperation with the Japanese. In English (JKB translation) it reads,

> What explains someone having been a non-cooperator? During the time of Dutch government all matters between Indonesia and Holland had the nature of disputing things of importance and necessity. If we wanted to go north, Holland wanted to go south, and if moving east, the Dutch wanted to go west. All matters and decisions during that time were under the control of the law of antithesis. With the presence of that law of antithesis, then the only one troublesome politic, concrete and not productive, is the politic of not working together: the politic of non-cooperation repeatedly announced by nationalists with spirited certainty. The politic of cooperation, yes, that is the politic that Great Indonesia reached for to work together with the Dutch—that is, productive politics, because it does not stand against the reality and reason of this world. And what about the current politics? Now there is a big line between Indonesia and Japan that is equally important and necessary. That big line now has the nature of synthesis. Japan intends to create Great Asia, as we wish only to create Great Asia. Japan intends to cleanse Great Asia of western imperialism, as we struggle for the same thing. Therefore, whereas before we had the politic of non-cooperation, now the flag will only sound the message of cooperation. We wanted to create Great Indonesia with a struggle to the end against Holland. Now we want to create Great Indonesia by working together with Japan.[6]

This is a reasoned argument, and it likely reflects his thinking at that time early in the occupation, but there was a critically important caveat: that the Japanese occupiers indeed shared Soekarno's vision of Indonesia Raya. History reveals they didn't, but Soekarno could not have known that, especially at that early juncture. His rational doubts motivated him to put contingencies in place. At the dawn of occupation, he asked key nationalists to go underground to prepare and wait for the order of open rebellion against the Japanese should such prove necessary. Those very early actions leave little doubt regarding Soekarno's willingness to sacrifice everything so far as Japan in Indonesia was concerned, for the ultimate goal of Indonesia Raya.

Intense and competing forces pressured Soekarno from all sides. While striving to sustain his nationalist bona fides and broad base of populist support, he nonetheless had to be careful not to displease the Japanese by even slightly undermining their absolute authority. Simultaneously he needed to maintain the loyalty of important and influential nationalists: not only his three associates at the top but also men like Soetan Sjahrir, a Minangkabau intellectual schooled in Holland. Soekarno and Hatta (Sjahrir was close with Hatta) met secretly with Sjahrir on the eve of Soekarno's first meeting with the new military occupation government. They urged Sjahrir to go underground to confront and resist the occupation should the Japanese become overtly hostile to Indonesian national identity and freedom. As it turned out, Sjahrir simply kept a low profile and readiness for a call to rebellion against the Japanese that never came. Sjahrir and his ready and able insurgents were yet another faction Soekarno had to keep in check and balance. Should those volatile factions act capriciously, all could be lost to overt Japanese military domination of the Indonesian territories provoked by the threat of open rebellion by 70 million inhabitants.

Ultimately Soekarno, Hatta, Dewantoro, Mansyoer, and men like Sjahrir were all on the same team and working toward the same objective—the Republic of Indonesia. They would struggle among themselves over precisely how to define the character of that republic, but for the time being the Pacific War was the stage on which their nationalist drama had to play. They did not yet have the national identity or credentials to be considered either Allied or Axis. They were a people struggling to obtain an independent national identity as yet undefined, and meanwhile playing the strategic cards dealt to them as best they could in their own vital and diverse interests. Certainly in the mind of Soekarno and most of his loyal followers, the Joyoboyo prophecies steeled their patience and resolve. Like most nationalists, Soekarno held his nose against Japanese deceits, arrogance, and cruelty, while keeping them on his side. All the while, he was getting on with the task of realizing the birth of the republic, whatever political stripes it ended up wearing.

The Republic

The Japanese finally allowed a formal conference on Indonesian independence in May 1945—by then firm in the knowledge that they had utterly nothing to lose. The Americans had invaded Okinawa, and their Nazi friends had surrendered unconditionally early that month. The Allied military might that had conquered the Nazis was already being repositioned in Guam, Formosa, and the Philippines in preparation for the planned onslaught against Honshu, the Japanese heartland. Independence for Indonesia became a building block for postwar revision of Imperial Japanese intent in their Pacific War— not colonial imperialists, but noble warriors fighting against colonial imperialism. The Japanese prodded the Indonesians to accomplish their independence before the Allies could arrive.

But the nationalists needed a political identity and a future-ensuring consensus on it. The conference on Indonesian independence in May 1945 was dubbed the Badan Penyelidikan Kemerdekaan Indonesia (Investigative Body for Indonesian Independence), or BPKI. The primary focus was on what, in very broad political brush strokes, a free Indonesia would look like.

A private struggle ensued between Soekarno and Hatta on that fundamental question in a geographic sense. Soekarno envisioned "Indonesia Raya" to include all of Borneo and the Malay Peninsula, that is, all of what is today Malaysia. Hatta, considering the claim and bounds indefensible politically or militarily, successfully reined in Soekarno's ambition to borders of the former Netherlands East Indies. Soekarno never quite gave up that dream, however. In 1962, without the benefit of Hatta's counsel and influence, Soekarno launched military attacks on Malaysian Borneo aimed at undoing the 1957 British creation of the independent nation of Malaya (renamed Malaysia when briefly incorporating Singapore, and not adjusted after reversal of that union by the government at Kuala Lumpur). Soekarno's Borneo campaign escalated through 1965 when it finally collapsed with his fall from power late that year.

In the 1945 BPKI, the secular nationalists put forth proposals defin-

New Reality

ing a secular democratic republic. The Javanese royalists pushed for a constitutional monarchy. Muslim leaders lobbied specific constitutional language acknowledging Islamic sharia'a as the law of the land—an Islamic republic. Hatta, himself a devout Muslim but also the primary intellectual and political muscle behind the secularist agenda, pointed to the example of secular Muslim Turkey and Mustafa Kemal Ataturk and dismissively painted the Islamic state as an anachronism. The debate in Jakarta thus raged.

Submerged and silent in the background—because the Japanese had no tolerance for them—were the formidable communist nationalists. Soekarno knew that when the Japanese exited, they too would demand that their powerful voice be heard.

When that voice did finally emerge in 1948, it was an angry and vengeful rebellion at Madiun in East Java, in the very midst of the republic's uncertain war for independence against the Dutch. One of the leaders of that uprising was Amir Sjarifuddin, who, like Soetan Sjahrir, had been asked by Soekarno at the dawn of occupation to go underground and resist the Japanese when and if called upon to do so. Moreover, Amir had accepted a large sum of money from the Dutch and covertly worked on their behalf during the occupation. The Japanese discovered he was a Dutch agent and captured him in 1943. They lawfully condemned him to execution, but Soekarno successfully pleaded that his life be spared. Amir, a highly educated man, became Soekarno's information minister (and Soetan Sjahrir the prime minister) in late 1945, an appointment perhaps aimed at placating the communists for their exclusion from the decisive BPKI. By some accounts (his friend Abu Hanifah, for example), Amir was not a true communist but one of opportunity (as with his agency of the Dutch during the occupation). Nonetheless, upon collapse of the communist rebellion at Madiun in 1948, Soekarno's troops executed Amir and many real communists. But surviving communists on Java, having deflected blame for the Madiun uprising upon a misguided splinter group, legally reorganized themselves under the protection of a sympathetic Soekarno. Their final rebellion and very bloody downfall, along with Soekarno's, would come in 1965 and 1966.

At the end of the BPKI in 1945, the secular nationalists won their secular democratic state, bringing the Islamists aboard with the concession that the president must be Muslim. The constitution of that year sealed the deal. It fell to Soekarno and his allies to pull all of the diverse cultures, languages, and religions across their archipelago into a single cohesive ideology. They did it with Pancasila, the five pillars of Indonesian national identity: nationalism (for everyone), humanitarianism (for everyone), democracy (for the secularists), social justice (for the communists), and belief in one god (for the Islamists, albeit specifying to their lasting dismay, any one god already worshipped in Indonesia). These attributions are grossly overly simplified, but they express the necessary balance aimed and hoped for.

Up to the present day, those planks of Indonesian national identity, including the 1945 constitution, stand firm despite a substantial and prolonged challenge from hardline Islamist factions. During the 1950s and 1960s Soekarno's troops crushed a well commanded and dangerous Darul Islam armed insurgency aimed at establishing an Islamic republic. Hardline Islamists view the "any one god" pillar of Pancasila—a decidedly secular principle—anathema to Islam and, as such, *haram*, or an affront to their beliefs. A band of hardline Indonesian jihadis fighting in Syria in 2014 posted a video imploring their countrymen to "discard Pancasila" and become true to Islam. Soekarno, and later Soeharto, acted deliberately and ruthlessly in suppressing Islamist-leaning ideologies they viewed as a threat to secularism and national unity.

Looking back, it is evident that Soekarno and Hatta succeeded spectacularly in walking a tightrope—the menacing Japanese on one side, and the fractious nationalists on the other. They remained true to the Boedi Oetomo and Youth Pledge vision of Indonesian national identity—a great, diverse secular republic. This came with tremendous costs, which Soekarno later freely admitted without actually specifying what those were.

The wholesale enslavement, torture, and slaughter of both ordinary and elite Indonesians by the Japanese occupier remained unutterable travesties for decades to come after the war. Among loyal and patriotic Indonesians this was especially taboo during the war of independence against the Dutch, when honestly facing the realities of what had occurred during the occupation could have been construed as treasonous. Postwar Indonesia seethed with injury and anger—against the Japanese, many of their Indonesian collaborators, the threatening Dutch and their sympathizers, and competing political ideologies within the fractious nationalist camp. Into that unstable mix the Dutch injected vicious propaganda of Japanese brutality in Indonesia to undermine the collaborating nationalists, both in the eyes of fellow Indonesians and the international powers weighing support of the nationalist cause. In so doing they forced the topic—including Mochtar's persecution—into a locked closet of dangerous truths. Dutch postwar aggression thus directly aided and abetted the burial of the truth of Japanese brutality in Indonesia.

Murder of Medicine

Indonesian physicians were, by colonial circumstance, also the flowers of Indonesian intellectualism. As such, the Japanese occupier feared and persecuted them. The execution of Dr. Roebini and his wife at Pontianak was just one of many firm demonstrations of inherent Japanese hostility toward people equipped to recognize and understand a hollow ruse when they saw one. This ability is the basis of the fearing and loathing of intellectuals by fascists everywhere. A developed intellect rarely accommodates the blind obedience and uncritical thinking so essential to the fascist agenda. The ruse of freedom for Indonesia was particularly thin but also crucial to Japanese Imperial designs for the East Indies. So the Japanese in Indonesia did what fascists typically do in dealing with such threats—they eliminated them.

A book published to celebrate the 125th anniversary of medical education in Indonesia in 1976 identifies Dr. Raden Soesilo (the prolific malariologist of Eijkman Institute fame, and also younger brother to one of the original Boedi Oetomo founders), Dr. Achmad Diponegoro (a direct descendant of the famous nineteenth-century exiled Javanese prince and rebellion leader Mustahar Diponegoro), Dr. Sunarjo, and Dr. Agusdjam (all STOVIA men) as victims of execution.[7] The exact justifications of these executions according to the Japanese are not known, except in the case of Raden Soesilo (implausibly speaking to American submarines surfacing in Indonesian rivers). We know that the physicians listed in that publication are not the only ones executed. There was no mention of Roebini, for example.

In his memoir of the Mochtar affair, Ali Hanafiah lists the names of nineteen doctors executed by the Japanese, including Roebini.[8]

Indonesian doctors and various other intellectuals at the time certainly felt under attack and considered themselves the focus of a Japanese effort to almost literally decapitate whatever Indonesian nationalist sentiments were not sufficiently under their control.

Abu Hanifah recalled a meeting at the time:

> I was present when Yamin [*Mohammad Yamin, a prominent Indo-nesian intellectual and friend to the Mochtar family*], an orator in his own right and one of our outstanding writers, and a couple of other friends were whispering that there existed a document, a Japanese plan to annihilate most of the top intellectuals of Indonesia. Only second-raters would be left who could be easily handled by the Japa-nese. The Japanese would then flood Indonesia with their own intel-lectuals. There must have been such a plan because so many top Indonesian intellectuals lost their lives during the Japanese occupa-tion for no reason at all.[9]

History proves Hanifah's suspicions well grounded. Gin gives a detailed accounting of the mass murder of civilians by the Japanese navy occupation forces in Borneo (Kalimantan) from 1942 to 1945.[10] The Japanese fabricated plots, using torture-induced confessions, and systematically executed hundreds in connection with each alleged plot. These included the "Haga Plot," the "Pontianak Incident," and the "Chinese Conspiracy" at Pontianak. Postwar investigation found that the occupiers decapitated 1,100 people at Mandor and Sungai Durian near Pontianak, accusing them of complicity in the Haga Plot and the Pontianak Incident. Gin mentions an unnamed Indo-nesian source in 1970 enumerating the number of victims of the Haga and Pontianak plots at 577 Indonesians (Malay race), 903 Chi-nese (Indonesians), 36 Europeans, and 18 "foreign Orientals." In the Chinese Conspiracy at Pontianak, between 170 and 200 ethnic Chi-nese Indonesians were beheaded.

According to Jun Yoshio, a Japanese civilian conducting wartime business in Borneo who was detained after the war, the above-named plots were fabricated in order to seize the belongings of wealthy residents. Hayashi Shuichi, a Japanese intelligence officer, testified after the war that he had been ordered to identify wealthy people, those who spoke Dutch (which all Indonesian doctors would be able to do), and "older people who remembered the Dutch administration too well." Those orders would net anyone of substance and influence. Gin closes with these words: "There is still a cache of untapped documents in the National Archives in Tokyo that might throw further light on this horrific episode, especially in regard to the existence of conspiracies and the Japanese motives to eliminate the local elites."

In an interview by the authors in 2010, Dr. Asikin Hanafiah and his sister Taty recalled a physician relative being murdered by the Japanese at Pontianak in 1944. The man's maid returned to Jakarta and told the family that he, along with dozens of others, were forced to the edge of a large pit and were shot by the Japanese. The townspeople, including the traumatized maid, had been forced to bear witness to the slaughter. No reason was known for his execution. The Japanese had come by his practice and taken him away without explanation. That man, and very many others like him, was executed for no other reason than a cultivated intellect.

Indonesians then, and today, considered the systematic murder of intellectuals and other influential Indonesians in Borneo a Japanese strategy aimed at resettling the huge island with its own citizens, completely displacing the indigenous people, except as needed for manual labor. Gin's recent article gives credence to this view, which has long been held among Indonesian families that lived through that terror.

The Japanese would have to apply a more subtle approach on the heavily populated islands of Java and Sumatra. Murdering most intellectuals in sight of the bulk of Indonesia's volatile masses was not feasible, so they had to be politically astute.

The community of medicine in the East Indies remained an object of keen and hostile interest to the Japanese authorities. They would certainly fear people who were intelligent enough to decipher the true intentions of the Japanese and who were respected enough by the masses to make their realization known. The STOVIA men and women lived in a terrifying uncertainty and a quite justifiable sense of the insecurity of their very lives. They watched the shadows of the sharks edging closer, bumping and taking down members of their professional family with every circling pass.

Casting Out the Dutch

The many thousands of Dutch in Batavia (and all across the archipelago) had been promptly rounded up by the Japanese and placed in prison camps in and around the city. Fathers and older sons were held apart from their mothers, daughters, and younger siblings. Some of the camps were simply cordoned-off blocks embedded within Jakarta, like the notorious Cideng camp in the Tanah Abang neighborhood. Homes that once housed a single family of five or six accommodated eighty or ninety living cheek to jowl in appalling filth, grossly insufficient rations, and rare and inadequate medical care. Dutch scientists and staff at the Eijkman Institute were all taken away, most probably landing at Cideng or a similar camp at Kramat, not far from the institute. We know Eijkman director W. K. Mertens was eventually interned at the Cimahi camp near Bandung, probably after being shuffled among three or four other camps as the Japanese constantly reorganized their placement. This was a typical experience for the male internees held on Java, while the women and children at Cideng remained at that site for the duration of the war.

The Japanese occupier did not engage in systematic deliberate murder of the civilian Dutch internees. They became an irrelevant logistical nuisance, and the Japanese very likely planned to repatriate them to Holland en masse after victory. Thanks to the enormous supply of "voluntary" labor from the Indonesian masses, few Dutch were subjected to the forced labor endured by many other civilian internees elsewhere in the empire of Japan. Many not surviving this captivity, as in the case of Mertens at Cimahi, often died as a consequence of gross neglect of nutrition and the most basic medical care for malaria, dengue fever, typhus, pellagra, diarrheal diseases, and beriberi. Pans Schomper recalled in his memoir as a teenage boy interred at Cimahi, "The hospital barracks were filled with men suffering hunger edema [beriberi] . . . they suffered from often unbearable stabbing pains in their feet." He continued later, "Dozens of corpses were carried out of the gate daily. The men died of exhaustion, bacillary dysentery and hunger edema. . . . The dead

were buried without any humanitarian concern in a cemetery outside camp. Every day we saw the same sight and we got used to it."[11]
Thus, though not spared cruelty, real misery, and murder by indifferent neglect, the extreme labor and summary executions that killed
so many elite Indonesians, Eurasians, ethnic Chinese, romusha, and
POWs were relatively rare among the interred Dutch.

The Indonesian staff left in place at the Eijkman, including Dr.
Mochtar, simply carried on after the Dutch were taken away. They
were largely unmolested by the Japanese, who seemed to have taken
no interest in their prestigious institute. Mochtar had succeeded
Mertens as director after his internment. We don't know how that
decision had been made or by whom, but it seems likely the Japanese did so in 1943 in conjunction with the reopening (and renaming
as Ika Dai Gaku) of the medical school and Mochtar's appointment
there as vice rector.

Eurasians

In 1942 Latifah Marzoeki was eleven years old. In a 2010 interview,
she recalled that her Dutch mother, Corrie (nee Spaanderman), and
Indonesian father, Dr. Marzoeki, were both Indonesian nationalists. She cited being a STOVIA family and nationalistic as insepara-
ble identities. She recalled socializing with "Oom" (Uncle) Mochtar
and "Tante" (Aunt) Hasnah. She described these terms of familiar-
ity as being used by all of the children of STOVIA graduates for the
colleagues of their parents. She clarified, "Not necessary that they
were really blood-related, but being Stovian was the same as being
family." She further explained that she called Mohammad Hatta
Oom because he was also like family, though not a Stovian. When
Hatta had been imprisoned in Holland, Corrie wrote to her Dutch
friends asking them to bring books and magazines for Oom Hatta.
In 1932 Marzoeki took Hatta to the beach at Pelabuhan Ratu on the
south coast of Java for a break from their labors, and Latifah provided a photo of the two men there.

As a racially mixed couple, the Marzoekis were sometimes treated
badly by the Dutch colonialists. The couple had abandoned race as
an important distinction, and Latifah recalled her parents meeting
the stares and whispers of their mixed arrangement with humor.

The Marzoekis also faced this mild sort of discrimination from Indonesian strangers, but their friends and neighbors welcomed Corrie into their diverse communities with genuine love. A group photo of a social gathering from the period shows Corrie and two other Dutch women among an Indonesian crowd. These were their friends and "family" of STOVIA graduates enjoying one of many such get-togethers. Mochtar and Siti Hasnah are present, with Marzoeki standing near him and Corrie seated near her. Ali Hanafiah and his wife are also present. We believe the Dutch woman seated near Corrie may be the wife of Dr. Suleiman Siregar, who may be the man in spectacles standing behind her—he was Marzoeki's employee and would not survive his arrest by the Kenpeitai in the Mochtar affair.

When asked if she understood that Eurasians were a favorite target of the Kenpeitai, Latifah seemed genuinely surprised. She pointed out that a distinction existed between Eurasians born to Dutch mothers and those with Dutch fathers. Indonesian men who married Dutch women were often, like Marzoeki, not only handsome and dashing but also highly educated. Conversely, most Indonesian women who married Dutch men in this era were not well educated or wealthy. Latifah warned of painting this trend too broadly—exceptions certainly occurred, acknowledging the blindness of true love to social station. The trend, though, affected the social possibilities for the children of these unions. The children of Dutch fathers gravitated to the higher station of the father and thus sought to be as Dutch as possible. Conversely, the children of Dutch mothers gravitated to the high standing of the accomplished Indonesian father. Those children, like Latifah and her two brothers, were unquestionably Indonesian in identity.

Latifah understood that the community of Indonesian Eurasians born to Dutch fathers suffered as targets of persecution by the Kenpeitai. Pausing to think about the Eurasian label and persecution, and the likelihood that those victims would be the Eurasian community of Dutch fathers, she surmised, "They would have been very pro-Dutch." She later amended that many such families also became ardent nationalists and did not deserve to be arbitrarily designated pro-Dutch, as the Kenpeitai did in ruthlessly persecuting them.

Corrie Marzoeki was not rounded up. Her prominent and connected Minangkabau STOVIA husband was able to protect her, but she took few chances to venture out. She spent most of the occupation years within the compound of her large home at Tanah Abang. Corrie's isolation was no Anne Frank–like hideout to avoid capture. The Japanese certainly knew she was there. They chose not to imprison her. They did not consider Corrie and women like her enough of a threat to risk alienating elite Indonesian communities with the arrest and imprisonment of the Dutch wives and mothers in their circles. Corrie's isolation represented caution against being mistakenly hauled away by a low-ranking Japanese trooper blind to such nuance. Dutch men married to Indonesian women, however, were hauled away and imprisoned. This would likely have driven the loyalties of their families toward the Dutch and Allied cause.

An Important Reminder

Latifah also warned the authors against painting the Japanese occupier too broadly. She recalled cordial relations with a Japanese civilian neighbor who shared the love of music in her family. (Corrie symbolized musical notes, la-ti-fah, in naming her daughter, an accomplished pianist throughout her long life.) She also described her father's relationship with the Japanese civilian mayor of Jakarta, his boss, as productive and mutually respectful. A Japanese civilian friend of the family, a Mr. Saito who had an American education, actually phoned the Marzoeki household on August 18, 1945, to congratulate them on the independence of their new nation. Saito implored them to go to the prison at once to demand the release of Dr. Marzoeki. She also recalled that the initially numerous Japanese civilians (most of them highly educated) were slowly whittled down, replaced with military men. The Imperial armed forces eventually assumed full control of all aspects of governance.

These recollections serve as an important reminder for readers of this book—while militarists and the military of Japan carried out a cruel and ruthless occupation, elite Japanese intellectuals brought a far more humane and productive approach to the occupation. The Japanese military eventually disposed of their civil agenda for Indonesia in favor of their own cruel approach. This sort of complexity exists in all societies; it did so in Imperial Japan and still does today in Japan. Though a minority, there are patriotic Japanese intellectuals today who tirelessly campaign—often risking social ostracism and even personal harm—for the Japanese nation to honestly face this dark chapter of their history. Some brave and enlightened Japanese lawyers, for example, heroically and generously volunteer their services to Chinese and Korean victims of the Japanese in suing the government on their behalf. Their kindred also existed in Imperial Japan during the war, even in territory brutally occupied by their militaristic countrymen. Latifah's testimony demonstrates this fact and wisely counsels us not to neglect such complexity.

EIJKMAN INSTITUTE, 1942–1944

As of 2014 only one person who had lived through the Mochtar affair as an alleged conspirator and Kenpeitai prisoner survives: Nani Kusumasudjana. She was discovered by Dr. Safarina Malik only through the coincidence that Nani's nephew, Dr. Tjohjono "Teddy" Gondhowiardjo, worked with the authors' colleagues at the Eijkman Institute in 2010. Arrangements were made, and on July 1, 2010, we traveled from Jakarta to Bogor to meet Ms. Nani, then eighty-seven years old. We met her at the elegant home of her son, Dr. Wahid, a distinguished and gracious man. Nani lived in this home. She was welcoming and curious about our visit. Her cordial and pretty twenty-something granddaughter snapped photographs.

In response to questions, Nani spoke softly, often pausing to remember and seemed to struggle to find the right words. But once she found the words, she spoke earnestly and plainly, sometimes lapsing into Dutch. Her memory carried her to where Dutch was often spoken. She had learned Bahasa Indonesia as a young woman, only after the Japanese had arrived. The Stovian household where she was raised had spoken Dutch.

Nani began working at the Eijkman Institute after the Japanese had arrived. She was unsure of the month, but it was 1942. She was just twenty-one and had been put to work in Dr. Mochtar's bacteriology laboratory. She recalled that her father, Dr. Kusumasudjana, had arranged the position.

She remained at the institute until her arrest by the Kenpeitai in mid-October 1944. Before her arrest, she could not recall any Japanese officers or civilians being at the institute. Though the Japanese had assumed daily and firm control of the adjacent medical school, they apparently had no interest in the research institute as a strategic or political asset. A photograph of the staff of the Eijkman Institute taken in 1943 shows several Japanese officers interspersed among them (fig. 22). One is seated next to Mochtar. Nani is standing directly behind another. We don't know who those officers were or why they sat for this photograph, but they apparently were not permanent fixtures at the institute.

Nani described Mochtar in those years as an extraordinarily kind and patient boss. When we showed her a portrait of a much younger Mochtar, likely taken after he completed his PhD at Amsterdam, she demanded, "Who is that?" When told that it depicted a younger Mochtar than she would remember, she remarked, "The Mochtar I knew had a much kinder face than that."

Asked what sort of man Mochtar had been, she thought for a few moments and then said simply, "*Dia orang baik sekali*" (he was a very good man). The word *baik* literally means "good," but in Indonesian, when referring to a person, it carries the additional connotations of kind, generous, honest, etc. It is deeper than simply "good," as is also sometimes true in English usage. She recalled him being a deeply intelligent man, but also being *tidak aneh,* or not strange or weird (as deeply intelligent people can be). Mochtar had been kind, intelligent, and easily understood as a man and thus approachable. She remembered his house at Cikini and his family being the focus of his life.

In her 1987 unpublished memoir Nani also recalled catching a rare glimpse of Mochtar in the Kenpeitai prison where she was held in late 1944. He was seated on a washboard used for torture (his legs were forced under him) as she was escorted past the open door. She described his demeanor as "calm and steadfast." Later still she saw him again in the brief moments before the Japanese guards put a cotton sack on his head for relocation within the prison (as was their routine). She remarked, "He held his head upright. He was definitely without sin." These glimpses sustained her will in her steadfast refusal to provide false testimony incriminating her boss, despite withering interrogations and the promise of survival and freedom.

Memoirs from Indonesians living under Japanese occupation reveal that the Japanese could not conceal the poor progress of their war. Through various streams, Indonesians understood that the Americans were seriously challenging the Japanese. Japan's stunning early victories did not translate into lasting success once they needed to sustain their hold on conquered territories. In 2010 Latifah Kodijat Marzoeki remembered hearing of the war's progress in whispers behind closed doors at home. She assumed that some people had access to forbidden radios and picked up reports. Having a radio was very dangerous, and its operator risked summary execution, but people swimming with sharks adapt to risk. The quasi-underground nationalist Soetan Sjahrir often visited the Marzoeki home during the war. Latifah remembered him as a fountain of information from the outside world. Looking back on his wealth of current information she said, "Yes, he must have had his own radio."

The importance of concealing the truth of the Japanese strategic posture may be illustrated by an event reported by Nani Kusumasudjana while held in Kenpeitai custody in late 1944. She described being interrogated by one Japanese man, when another burst into the room shouting some urgent piece of news. They breathlessly repeated the amazing news for her in Indonesian language—the Japanese navy had utterly destroyed the American navy in an epic battle in the Pacific Ocean. This was a ploy aimed at convincing Nani she would be living under Japanese rule for some time and that she should cooperate more fully with them to ensure her future. She declared, knowing with certainty at the time, that it was a preposterous bluff and lie.

Indeed the scale of military disasters stalking Imperial Japan in their war were epic and, by late 1944, irreversible. The abrupt halt of Japan's Pacific sweep at the Battle of the Coral Sea in mid-1942 (losing two aircraft carriers to heavy damage) was swiftly followed by the breathtaking losses suffered by the Japanese at the sea battle of Midway, with four precious aircraft carriers and a cruiser destroyed and sunk. The Americans lost a single aircraft carrier, the *Yorktown*, and a mere destroyer. During the island campaign at Guadalcanal, the naval battles at Iron Bottom Sound deepened their losses and their ability to sustain or evacuate troops on that island, all of whom were ultimately killed or captured, the latter a very small minority.

The Australians and the Americans halted the Japanese southerly push for Port Moresby on the bloody Kokoda trail across the mountainous spine of New Guinea. MacArthur's amphibious march up the north coast of New Guinea reached the Netherlands East Indies eastern outpost of Hollandia (now called Jayapura in Indonesian Papua) in April 1944; a monument stands today at the site of his headquarters on a hilltop overlooking Lake Sentani. Hollandia became a logistical staging area for the planned invasion of the Philippines. Residents of modern Jayapura recalled their enormous harbor and bay being so full of ships that it seemed one could walk all of the way across it. Neighborhoods in that city today retain names of that era: near the city center is "APO" where the military post office had operated, and "Base G" is a beach where one of the Allied landings occurred. Other neighborhoods are identified as "Dock 2" or "Dock 5" where today docks no longer stand.

MacArthur would push out from Hollandia and take hold of the Indonesian islands of Halmahera and Morotai to the west of New Guinea, after ferocious battles at Wakde, Biak, and Noemfoor along that coast. American bomber sorties from bases at Biak and Morotai seriously harassed Japanese shipping and outposts all across central and eastern Indonesia. American submarines prowled the Java and South China Seas, severely punishing Japanese supply and logistics. The evidence of Allied military activity along the eastern Indonesian archipelago would have elevated Japanese anxiety concerning an amphibious assault of scale in the East Indies. The same would also raise bright hope in Indonesians of the brevity of Japanese rule promised in *Joyoboyo Pralembang*.

The Americans paused at Halmahera and Morotai and then turned northward, toward the Philippines, rather than challenge Japanese possession of the rest of the East Indies. MacArthur had his eyes on his beloved Philippines and his promise to return after his narrow escape by patrol boat and submarine from Corregidor in early 1942. American war strategy aimed for the Japanese mainland to the north and deliberately avoided enclaves of Japanese might along the way. MacArthur bypassing the Japanese strongholds in the East Indies was in keeping with his conduct of the war up to that point. For example, MacArthur's forces had simply slipped around the 110,000 Japanese troops entrenched at Rabaul, New Guinea. The Americans bombed their threatening gear out of commission and the U.S. Navy cordoned off the island, depriving them of resupply. Among the massive concentration of Japanese troops on that island, most died of a cruelly imposed starvation; the survivors had resorted to cannibalism.

The Japanese garrison at Rabaul had been rendered militarily irrelevant by simply sailing past it. The same would be true of the Japanese all throughout Southeast Asia, except the Philippines (and Adm. Chester Nimitz had vigorously advocated bypassing it as well). Liberation of the East Indies and the rest of Southeast Asia, Allied strategy dictated, would come with the fall of Tokyo. The American military dagger aimed squarely for that target and turned its back on the Indonesian archipelago in early 1945. The Japanese in the East Indies at the time, however, could not know this. On Java and elsewhere, they prepared and braced for an invasion and combat that would never materialize.

Dr. Asikin Hanafiah recalled a conversation in 1943. Oom Mochtar sat him down and earnestly instructed him to study English, which he did and now speaks with fluent ease. Mochtar explained to his nephew that the Japanese would lose the war to the Americans and that speaking English would become a key advantage to him. Listening to Asikin's superb English and knowing its origins, one cannot help but feel Mochtar's presence.

Mochtar saw Allied victory over the horizon, both in Europe and Asia. His Kenpeitai captors would later say of Mochtar to one of his fellow prisoners, "If we cut open the stomach of Mochtar we would find an American flag."

Ironically, the American bypass of Java and the defeat of Imperial Japan spelled Mochtar's doom. The occupier could not permit him to survive to meet inquisitive Allied tribunal prosecutors.

Mochtar's family would receive the devastating news that their son Baharsjah had passed away in his home at Leiden in the Netherlands on February 21, 1944. The cause of death was reported as pulmonary tuberculosis, but most Dutch know the winter of 1944 under Nazi occupation as the "winter of hunger." Baharsjah did not survive those rigors. No direct record of when the Mochtars learned of this tragic news is known. However, Nani Kusumasudjana recalled in 2010 that Mochtar knew of his son's death before being arrested by the Kenpeitai. She remembered the deep trauma this news inflicted on her boss some months before he was taken away.

While imprisoned, Mochtar must have worried deeply about Siti Hasnah, home alone, mourning Baharsjah and anxious about her sole surviving son, Imramsjah, alone and still trapped in Holland. His own situation would, of course, compound her deep anxiety and his worry for her. Mochtar had months to contemplate his family and his own fate. He surely understood his improbable survival depended upon an Allied invasion of Java. It would have seemed perfectly plausible to him. He knew the Allies had brought enormous resources to bear in shrinking the Japanese Empire. Australia remained their base in the western Pacific sphere, and they held all of New Guinea. Could they not launch an invasion force against the isolated Japanese fortress on Java, as they had done at Normandy in June 1944? Cut off from information by his arrest and isolation in October 1944, he could not have known this as a vain hope. Indeed, Nani Kusumasudjana described in her memoir a rare Allied aerial bombing of Jakarta while she was imprisoned (October to November 1944), with the planes flying low directly over the prison. Mochtar likely held out some hope for his survival up to the moment they removed that cotton sack from his head at the execution ground at Ancol.

EIGHT

Klender

Invisible Holocaust

The overt murders of intellectual and financial elites in Indonesia by the Japanese, along with the racially motivated killing of Eurasians and Chinese and the murder by neglect of internees and prisoners of war, may be counted in the many tens of thousands. As horrific as all of these losses may be, when weighed against those of the romusha, they pale in comparison. Estimates of the numbers recruited and taken away range between 4 and 10 million. The precise number cannot be known, but by almost any reasoned and evidence-informed estimate it seems likely that several million did not survive that cruel captivity.

The romusha were also exported beyond Indonesia, principally to Thailand and Burma. The romusha slaves in those countries included Malaysians, Burmese, Chinese, and Vietnamese, in addition to Allied POWs. The famous Hollywood film of the fictional story *Bridge over the River Kwai* (1957) inaccurately depicts POWs at work in the absence of these romusha and almost completely fails at conveying the true severity of that captivity. The producers of that film hinted at the romusha in the script by casting Asian women as sympathetic (and sex interest) co-conspirators and having the women complain that the Japanese had taken their men away. Starving, beaten, and diseased men forced to work in tropical heat on pain of death would unlikely exhibit defiance of any sort, much less conspire to patriotically slow down the Japanese war machine by ingenious means. That would require a degree of humane treatment that, by all accounts, was entirely absent from forced labor sites all across Southeast Asia. The POWs and romusha were wholly consumed by a daily struggle for personal survival in a hellish captivity of starvation, forced labor, routine brutality, summary executions, and a withering climate of endemic tropical diseases. That film and its popularity directly contributed to the invisibility of the holocaust of unimaginably brutal forced labor by the Imperial Japanese during the Pacific War.

The dispensing of the romusha from that movie script effectively represents their treatment in our collective awareness of the history of the Pacific War, which, especially in the West, tends to look exclusively at the experiences of Allied military men in that struggle. Ignorance of or indifference to the epic suffering and slaughter of the romusha cries for moral and historic redress.

For the millions of romusha held in camps within Indonesia, documentation of their death or survival doesn't exist. Many of these undoubtedly did survive beyond the reach of systems to count them. Still others likely resettled where liberated, in Indonesia or abroad. It is known, for example, that modest numbers of Indonesian romusha became Thai nationals after the war. However, the estimated number of survivors never approached that of the men taken. Firm counts of the Indonesian romusha dead indicate several hundred thousand, but *firm* should not be misconstrued as even nearly complete or somehow authoritative. The vast numbers of wholly unaccounted men must also be weighed. Shigeru Sato reported that the Soekarno government of Indonesia demanded $10 billion from the government of Japan for reparation against their estimate of the loss of 4 million lives under the romusha program.[1] The Japanese government rejected the claim, citing a lack of evidence, as they had done repeatedly in the instance of the "Comfort Women." The government of Japan did formally apologize to those women in the 1990s, but Japanese nationalists today campaign for the withdrawal of that apology, citing the lack of evidence.

Romusha survivors from the many hundreds of work sites all across the Japanese Empire described essentially similar experiences. They had been held captive at gunpoint in guarded compounds, given grossly inadequate rations, no medical attention whatsoever, forced to perform backbreaking labor, routinely beaten for the slightest offense, and summarily executed for insubordination, theft, or attempted escape. Infections like malaria, dengue, typhus, and enteric diseases went untreated, as did serious nutritional deficiencies like beriberi and scurvy. Each of these maladies came with very high rates of mortality. The best a romusha could hope for was to be treated as a slave and thus at least be valued as property. More often, however, their treatment reflected a view of their being disposable. The supply of romusha must have seemed limitless to their Japanese keepers. Like their Allied POW brethren, many of them could not and would not survive this sort of inhumane captivity. Nine out of every ten Allied POW deaths in all theaters of World War II occurred at the hands of Japanese captors.

Almost no one outside of Indonesia has ever heard about the romusha and their plight, a fact which speaks to the invisibility of these millions of victims of slavery and murder. *Romusha* is a Japanese word for "unskilled laborer," but any Indonesian today understands it as "slave laborer." The word appears in English dictionaries of the Indonesian language (e.g., "local forced laborers during the Japanese occupation of Indonesia").[2]

How can the murder of several million people escape notice? Even just the relatively well documented losses of the very small minority of romusha exported beyond Indonesia yields a number of dead approximating the number of Indonesians carried away in the 2004 Asian tsunami at Aceh: about 220,000 souls. The broader estimates reside in the numerical neighborhood of those systematically slaughtered by the Nazis: Jews, gypsies, homosexuals, and the mentally or genetically impaired. Those victims did not suffer the further and deeper injustice of invisibility to our collective memory.

The Dutch cemetery at Cimahi near Bandung offers further evidence of that injustice for the romusha dead. There stands a modest monument to the sinking of the cargo ship *Junyu Maru* in 1944. Almost no one would recognize that ship's name and put it into the same league with, for example, the sinking of the *Titanic*. Post explains that the *Junyu Maru* sinking is the worst shipping tragedy of all time up to the present day.[3] A known 5,620 lives were lost, over three times as many as the 1,490 who perished on the *Titanic*. Virtually all of the *Junyu Maru* dead were POWs and romusha.

The British submarine *Tradewind* out of Sri Lanka was patrolling the western Sumatra coast on September 17, 1944. The *Junyu Maru* was a dozen miles from the coast, almost exactly halfway between Padang and Bengkulu. At 3:51 p.m. at a range of 1,800 yards *Tradewind* fired the first of two torpedoes into the *Junyu Maru*. The submarine crew could not have known of her human cargo. Of the 2,200 Allied POWs, 680 survived the sinking (69 percent mortality). Among the 4,200 romusha aboard, only 200 are believed to have survived (95 percent mortality). The survivors of the *Junyu Maru* disaster were later deposited at their original destination, the notoriously lethal Pekanbaru rail line construction in Sumatra. According to Willem Wanrooy, a Dutch POW survivor of both the sinking and the rail project, 95 POWs from the *Junyu Maru* also survived that project (86 percent mortality at the rail line, and 96 percent mortality overall).[4] Wanrooy declares that none of the 200 romusha who survived the *Junyu Maru* sinking saw the completion of the Pekanbaru rail project, which occurred the day before the Japanese surrender on August 14, 1945. The commander of the Pekanbaru rail project, Capt. Miyazaki Ryohei, overseeing the deaths of many thousands of romusha and POWs, was tried, convicted, and executed by Allied war tribunal. He is another heroic "divinity" honored at Yasukuni.

Gotong Royong

Understanding why the Indonesian romusha dead are forgotten lies in grasping the complex political relationship between the occupier and the occupied in Indonesia and of the political and military landscape of Indonesia and all of East Asia after the war. That clarity, in turn, informs our quest to understand the murder of Achmad Mochtar.

In whatever lands the Japanese occupied, they put local people, POWs, and interned civilians to work at gunpoint in the heavy task of making their new holdings militarily suitable. That typically meant building installations or industries in direct support of their military's aims and needs, like mining raw materials, constructing airfields, barracks, docks, railroads, and other infrastructural needs.

As General Imamura patiently explained to Soekarno, the fate of

Indonesia was in the hands of the emperor, and this matter would not be decided until after the war.[5] The message to Soekarno was clear: the quicker we win the war, the quicker you win independence, and the more you please the emperor, the more likely he is to view your independence favorably. Soekarno came to view direct support of the Japanese war effort as direct support of Indonesian independence. As surely connived by the Japanese, he rallied his loyal masses to this cause.

Gotong royong is an Indonesian expression that means to pull together voluntarily and cooperatively to achieve something for the common good. It can be applied to a massive national effort or a task as simple as refurbishing a local school. Soekarno harnessed the gotong royong spirit in rallying his people to aid the Japanese war effort and thereby their own freedom and independence.

Thus the Japanese cloaked the practice of forced labor in Indonesia as a voluntary, patriotic service to a common and worthy cause. Numerous Japanese propaganda posters and films from the era of occupation affirm this. The charade served the political aims of both the Japanese and the nationalists: a win-win for leaders. The Japanese obtained a vast pool of laborers in support of their military objectives, and Soekarno won the support of the Japanese in his leadership position, in addition to deposits in the emperor's bank of goodwill for the granting of independence. In this high exchange, the romusha conscripts obtained hellish bondage to beastly masters willing to drive them to their deaths.

A story recounted in 2013 by Djumina, the ninety-five-year-old grandmother of Ms. Lenny Ekawati (a scientist who works at the Eijkman Institute) may be considered perhaps a typical experience of the romusha program at the countless villages that supplied the men. She was living at Gunung Kidul near Yogjakarta, central Java, in late 1943 when her brother, the village leader, made a call for romusha volunteers. The men were implored to do their duty in support of nationhood and independence. They were promised decent food, housing, and work, along with a cash bonus for signing up. Families that refused to contribute volunteers faced loss of government subsidies of foodstuffs (during a time of great hunger), but most refused to give up their young men. Six men in that village did volunteer and received a cash bonus, which they left with their families and their intact flow of government ration subsidies. Five of those men would never return, their fates left unreported to the families. One man did return after the war, but according to Djumina he had been so traumatized by what he experienced that he was psychologically ruined for the remainder of his life.

Soekarno's memoirs acknowledge most of this, and in all fairness he had few options available to him. The Japanese controlled the archipelago with guns, swords, and an unflinching willingness to use them. The moment Soekarno became less useful, or became a threat, he would have been removed and replaced with a more pliant leader. This would have been a hard sell to the Indonesian masses and a very risky gambit for the Japanese, but they had demonstrated no aversion to harshness, coercion, or risky gambits. Soekarno certainly understood this, too, and explicitly expressed this sense of vulnerability during the war.

The Japanese in Indonesia, as they had consistently demonstrated in all of their other new holdings, would have certainly taken the laborers without the consent of local leaders. The charade of Indonesian romusha volunteerism greatly simplified and mitigated the risk of rebellion in implementing the task, but it mattered only in the relationship between the leaders of the occupied and occupier. On the ground, where the labor occurred, volunteerism ceased to matter and was completely discarded in favor of the efficiency of brutal coercion.

Among young Indonesian women similarly recruited to serve in support of Japanese troops in various domestic and technical capacities, the charade of volunteerism also vanished when they found themselves sexually enslaved by the Japanese occupier. This particularly barbaric dimension of the occupation, though publically aired in other formerly Japanese-occupied nations, has not been adequately addressed in the Indonesian context. Abu Hanifah acknowledged the practice like this: "And then there were thousands of young women and girls from the villages sent out ostensibly to serve as nurses at the front to help the wounded, brave Japanese soldiers back to health again. These poor girls disappeared mostly in the camp brothels of the Japanese armies."[6] He also describes a young pretty Eurasian woman brought to his clinic for medical attention after being abused by Japanese officers at a party the night before. She had dozens of burns caused by cigarettes. Hanifah recalled, "The burns were worst on her lower body, particularly on her thighs, her buttocks, her calves, and even her genitals. . . . What sadists I thought. And I felt a mad rage rising in me because I was so powerless."[7] William Bradley Horton describes evidence suggesting a complex mix of coercion and persuasion in the brothels servicing Japanese troops.[8]

A cultural or political reluctance to acknowledge the sexual enslavement of Indonesian women by the Japanese should not be construed as evidence of having not occurred. To borrow a scientific axiom: the absence of evidence is not evidence of absence. The occupier certainly sexually exploited Indonesian women, but an exploration of the scale and reach of that travesty exceeds the scope of this book.

Hard Enough

The romusha men often worked on the same sites as Allied POWs and were in equally dire straits with regard to their treatment by the Japanese captors. They faced hellish labor, starvation, disease, and physical brutality. Those who faltered in work, obedience, or display of overt subordination to their keepers would not survive.

At one site within Indonesia, the romusha appeared to have had slightly more liberties than the POWs. William E. Johns, gunnery officer on the HMS *Exeter*, which was sunk in the Battle of Java Sea in February 1942, was imprisoned at Makassar in the southern Celebes. At one point he was transferred to work a nickel mine at Pamalla near Kendari in southeastern Celebes (today called Sulawesi). He described his impression of the romusha crews working the same mine:

> By this time, we had become friendly with the forced laborers from Java, and what little money we had we gave to them and asked them to buy food of any kind for us. This they would do, and some mornings, guided by stones that were thrown by them, we would slide away to a bush or clump of growth to find perhaps a bunch of bananas or some Java sugar. Life was hard enough for those Indonesians, yet they helped us, and many a POW who survived owes his life to the little extras they bought for us in the native compound where they lived.[9]

When starving, disease-ridden, and almost daily beaten POWs describe someone else's condition as "hard enough," it speaks to the severities endured by the Indonesian "volunteers." This touching tribute to their kindness and courage also hints at the enormous alienation from the Japanese "big brother" that romusha must have quickly acquired. The Japanese aggressively prohibited feeding POWs. Starvation was a means of keeping them docile and in an almost biologically enforced state of subordination.

Johns describes a POW caught smuggling a fruit in from a work party outside the gates and very nearly being beheaded as a consequence. Instead, he was beaten to within an inch of his life. The romusha understood that feeding the POWs carried a lethal risk. At least at Pamalla, the romusha seem to have viewed the Allied POWs as fellow prisoners with a mutual tormentor and enemy: their Japanese captors. Men struggling to survive against a force that mutually threatens their lives form bonds of brotherhood. In Johns's testimony we can see this from both the POWs and the romusha slaves.

The Cruelest Hoax

The political dimension of Japanese management of the romusha program has been explained, where such cooperation served to sustain good relationships among leaders of occupied and occupier. Providing political cover to the supportive Indonesian leaders required decent treatment of the romusha when in sight of the Indonesian masses on Java. By most accounts this indeed occurred. Soekarno and other leaders thus faced no serious challenge or firm doubts regarding their sponsorship of the romusha program during its active implementation. The spirit of gotong royong, so far as most ordinary Indonesians could see, engaged the organizational skills and logistical resources of the occupier in harnessing labor aimed at the common cause of independence and freedom. Indonesians could view the romusha as being humanely managed with decent housing, clothing, meals, and even expert medical care in preparation for their service to the nation and empire at remote sites. Such is the message repeatedly delivered in Japanese propaganda of that period and place.

Some romusha were assigned to the relatively few work sites on

Java. The island already had substantial standing infrastructure when the Japanese arrived. At those sites in plain view of many Indonesians, the Japanese were careful to sustain the illusion of humane treatment. One Japanese propaganda photograph shows Soekarno wearing outdoor kit overseeing a vast labor effort behind him. Apart from the obvious value of maintaining the ruse of humanity and common cause, as a practical matter, romusha on Java could simply bolt from such work sites and completely vanish into the sea of Javanese people surrounding them. Sato explains the relative lack of violence against romusha on Java in this context.[10]

An important exception on Java was the Banten rail line built at Cikotak in a remote mining district in West Java detailed in the history by H. A. Poeze. Conditions for the romusha here were as hellish as anywhere, and an estimated 90,000 were killed. A Eurasian Indonesian personnel manager at that location (cited in Poeze's chapter) recounted that

> the ruthless occupier, who fagged us out and allowed us not a single free day, was guilty of the death daily of dozens of romusha, who were made to do slave labor, received very bad and insufficient food and almost no medical treatment. Those weakened romusha had practically no resistance to disease, and countless numbers fell victim to malaria. The Japanese did not care what happened to them; after all there was a new supply of romushas every week.[11]

This testimony contradicts that of a senior Javanese romusha overseer who described decent treatment and the deaths of only 3 of his 1,000-man workforce at the same location and time. Its veracity is doubtful.

Another Javanese witness at this site, Sutawinangun, cited in Poeze's chapter, affirms the horrors that occurred. He described recruitment under false pretexts and patriotic appeals, along with promises of good working conditions and pay. He recalled,

> But after they had reached their designated location their hopes for a happy existence instantly vanished when they saw the romusha who had arrived earlier . . . were as emaciated as skeletons. . . . Day and night there was heavy work, with no consideration of the scorching

sun, the heavy rain, or the hard wind that ravaged the laborers . . .
not a few dropped dead and lay in the middle of a field in the heat of
the sun, or next to a heap of earth they had dug out for themselves.
Others died on the banks of a river, of thirst, whilst they crawled
towards it in search of water. . . . Still others died while resting under
a tree. . . . All of this had become commonplace; nobody was disturbed by it or mourned it.[12]

The cruel ruse of the Japanese thus played out even on Java itself,
albeit still far from the eyes of the political elite. Young men were
recruited, shipped out, and promptly worked to death by the thousands. Survivors of the Banten rail project, within a three-day hike of
Jakarta, must have relayed the horrors they experienced. The nationalists must have had some inkling of the truth. Soekarno certainly
hints at such awareness in his 1965 autobiography, but pointed to
wartime sacrifices for the common cause of freedom and independence from the white imperialists.[13]

We know the Japanese mitigated the political risks to the nationalist leaders with propaganda that included sites like the Klender
transit camp outside Jakarta. There they lavished the romusha with
relatively generous food, medical care, and humane treatment.

A Javanese father seeing such an operation would not hesitate
to urge his son to enlist and would have no reason to question the
encouragement (and financial incentives) to do so heard emphatically
from the political elite. The relative extremes of kindness shown to
the romusha at sites like Klender, and the rest of the patriotic propaganda that put people in it, may thus be recognized as the most grotesque of inhumanities—the Japanese managed the romusha young
men (and those who cared about them, including their political leaders) much as a herder manages domesticated livestock, where slaughter must occur beyond sight of the flock to avoid grasp of their own
fate. The flock sees only a caring herder, until selected individuals
ultimately meet the butcher.

Lifting the Veil

The cynical golden rule in military cultures everywhere is "never
volunteer." It is based on the belief that commanders are less com-

mitted to one's personal welfare than they are to their own advancement. This rule finds few better expressions than in the romusha program in occupied Indonesia. An examination of the recruitment or impressment of romusha is important to the Mochtar affair and requires some consideration.

Soekarno's difficult position with the Japanese in the romusha context has been explained. The Japanese recognized his immense and loyal following. They exploited his charismatic nature to obtain the laborers they required. Soekarno came to be widely viewed, then and now, as the chief recruiter of romusha for the Japanese. He undertook the endeavor energetically, doing so in the firm belief he was both helping the Japanese to physically repel the colonialists and making goodwill deposits ensuring the emperor's favorable decision on independence. The recruitment campaigns, and the consequences, were another heavy burden to bear in winning Indonesia Raya. Soekarno frequently traveled around Java during the war, cementing his alliances and loyalties among local leaders and imploring them to provide romusha to the Japanese. In September 1944 Soekarno and many other elites volunteered as romusha for one week to boost flagging recruitment numbers.[14]

Soekarno was frank about his leading role in recruiting romusha long after the war. In *Soekarno: An Autobiography*, he described a meeting with medical students during the war (stoked by a critic of Soekarno, Soetan Sjahrir). They angrily challenged Soekarno's dealings with the Japanese, especially in delivering the romusha into their hands. He recounted his response to them as follows:

> There are casualties in every war. A Commander-in-Chief's job is to win the war even if it means losing a few battles on the way. If I must sacrifice thousands to save millions, I will. We are in a struggle for survival. As leader of this country, I cannot afford the luxury of sensitivity.
>
> My lot is to keep the Japanese believing I am swaying the masses to their aid. Otherwise, they will remove me, and we are now on the brink of what we've been fighting for all our lives. At all costs I must stay in this position. Only I can keep the pressure on Japan and I can keep the lid on Indonesia—until the time is right.[15]

His response to the queries of Cindy Adams on this issue was even more stark. "In fact, it was I, Sukarno, who sent them to work. Yes, it was I. I shipped them to their deaths. Yes, yes, yes, I am the one. . . . It was horrible, hopeless. And it was I who gave them to the Japanese. Sounds terrible, doesn't it? . . . Nobody likes the ugly truth."[16]

By his own stunningly honest words Soekarno explained both his role and the political stake he held in the romusha program. He also expressed understanding of the hazards and hardships of the romusha. He viewed them, effectively, as soldiers—lost in cause to the nation.

A newspaper clipping from soon after the war—propaganda inspired by the Dutch seeking to undermine Soekarno's political base—assigned responsibility to Soekarno for the suffering of the romusha. It showed a photograph of three filthy and skeletal romusha liberated by MacArthur's troops at Noemfoor in northwestern Dutch New Guinea. The article explained that of 1,600 romusha sent to the site, only 251 survived some months later, the balance of 1,349 dying of starvation, disease, beatings, and beheadings. The article was provocatively addressed to Soekarno. It asked him how it felt to see what he had done. This sort of poison issued by those striving to reassert colonial domain effectively walled off the topic for the nationalists.

Though it is enemy propaganda, the article nonetheless illustrates Soekarno's political vulnerability regarding the revelation of the truth of the romusha program after the war. And Soekarno was not alone in this culpability. In addition to countless village leaders all across Java, like Djumina's brother at Gunung Kidul, prominent Indonesians with solid nationalist credentials shared in the responsibility for the recruitment and impressment of the romusha.

Among many others, Koesoemo Oetoyo stands out by his direct link to the camp at Klender. This man from Semarang in central Java held senior leadership positions both in the Dutch colonial government (he was the regent of Jepara, Central Java, from 1905 to 1925) and the nationalist movement. He served as chairman of Boedi Oetomo (the STOVIA-founded national identity movement) from 1926 to 1936. During the Japanese occupation he held a senior post in the Department of Internal Affairs that included the task of collecting and administering the romusha. This included, according to the *Encyclopedia of Indonesia in the Pacific War*, "looking after the romusha stopping over in Jakarta [the Klender camp] during their transit on their way to places outside Java."[17]

The Japanese installed the highly respected Oetoyo as the Indonesian responsible for the welfare of the romusha at the Klender camp. Historians consider that camp to have been a model or showcase facility—physical propaganda. In hindsight such may be recognized as part and parcel of the broader cruel ruse. Visiting the camp, as we presume he did, Oetoyo would have perceived few concerns for his charges or his political base by taking responsibility for their welfare.

This outlook would radically change in early August 1944 when nine hundred romusha corpses littered that model camp. Assigning blame for the deaths became a high stakes political matter. The Japanese scientists responsible had inadvertently lifted the veil concealing Japanese cruelty. The larger flock had glimpsed the slaughterhouse.

Scene of the Crime

The romusha camp at the village of Klender lay between Jakarta and the town of Bekasi a few miles to the east. A railhead there connected lines from Java to the Jakarta seaport at Tanjung Priok. In 1944 Klender was little more than rice paddies and the humble homes of farmers. Today it is an urbanized piece of metropolitan Jakarta. The population of Jakarta in 1944 was about 200,000, and today the larger metropolitan area stands at about 18 million.

We do not know exactly what the romusha camp at Klender looked like or its precise location, other than it was near the rail line. No photos have yet been discovered. Nonetheless, from eyewitness descriptions we can surmise that it was a fenced compound with gates controlled by Japanese sentries. Given its relatively rural location, it may have been a purpose-built new construction. The Klender camp was a transit station used by successive waves of romusha cohorts. The romusha were likely drilled in military formation and marching; Indonesian recruits into the civil service of various government ministries do so routinely even today. The intent of such drilling is not militarism but cohesion among people coming together and engaging in a shared endeavor. It is the spirit of gotong royong.

The model status of the camp at Klender, due to its proximity to almost every important Indonesian nationalist, likely ensured a wholesome environment and relatively friendly Japanese sentries and camp officers. We know medical care was routinely provided, both preventive medicine and acute care. Nonetheless, few of the romusha volunteered for even this sham of humane treatment. Abu Hanifah recalled seeing well-educated young men in a group of romusha he had the duty to examine medically. Curious, he asked those young men why they had volunteered. They explained they had not volunteered at all.[18] They were summoned by village heads and then taken away by Japanese soldiers. According to sources surveyed by the *Encyclopedia of Indonesia in the Pacific War*, only about 20 percent of romusha willingly volunteered.[19]

Regardless of the individual circumstances of their recruitment, the young romusha at Klender found themselves thrown together as a group. There would have been clutches of them from the same village, and many of those would have known one another since birth. But like all groups of people of the same young age, eating the same food, sleeping in the same buildings, and headed for the same unknown, they formed new friendships fast. They would have been as young as fifteen and as old as forty. Among the few actual volunteers, they would have had few prospects at home except familiar paddies. Most romusha had probably not previously ventured more than fifty kilometers from where they had been born, and would likely have anticipated the journey to unknown destinations elsewhere in the vast empire of Japan with a sense of anxious adventure. Most would have been unaware of the extreme cruelty and hardship awaiting them, had they survived the experiment to be performed on them.

Their preparations for service to the empire and their country included medical screening and vaccinations. They would have been ordered to muster in ranks by the Indonesian camp bosses who were, in turn, managed by relatively kindly disposed Japanese military overseers. They would have been militarily drilled and trained to do so. A roll call of the ordered ranks would have been made, with all present or accounted for. Groups would have been lined up in orderly fashion and marched in turn to where the doctors waited. They would have been told to obey the doctors, who would give them an injection that would keep them healthy in their new, important duties.

Most of them would be unfamiliar with doctors and injections. There would have been trepidation and mild teasing of the conspicuously fearful to break the tension as they witnessed the big needles going into arms. They would have laughed nervously at the reflexive wincing of the injected. Later they would have compared their welts and complained of the soreness with good humor. It would have seemed part of the adventure in which they were all bound together.

The two doctors supervising and actually doing most of the injections were STOVIA men, Dr. Marah Achmad Arief and Dr. Suleiman Siregar. They were from the municipal health service of Jakarta. Their boss, Dr. Marzoeki, had received orders from the Japanese military to provide this manpower. They departed for the site with nothing more than their medical bags, having been informed that all else would be provided, including the vaccines (according to Dr. Marzoeki's notes in the memoirs of his daughter, Latifah). Testimony provides no more than this. The men apparently went to Klender, accepted the vaccination materials from the Japanese camp masters, and proceeded with the formidable task of vaccinating hundreds of romusha. Neither Arief nor Suleiman would survive arrest by the Kenpeitai a few months later. No testimony from them survives, unless the Kenpeitai record of their testimony under torture rests in dusty Japanese government archives.

The available recorded testimony skips forward to early August 1944. It comes from Dr. Bahder Djohan as recorded in the memoir of the Klender episode by Dr. Ali Hanafiah, and was also captured by Theodore Friend in a 1968 interview of Bahder Djohan.[20] Djohan who went on to a distinguished career that included two terms as the minister of education, science, and culture and as president of the University of Indonesia.[21] The same account appears in the biography of Djohan assembled by a team of Indonesian authors and published in 1980.[22]

Djohan's testimony tells us that the phone rang at the Ika Dai Gaku hospital (formerly Central Hospital) at Weltevreden in Jakarta (today Cipto Mangunkusumo Hospital in Salemba) at 9 a.m. Sunday. It was a frantic phone call from Klender reporting many dozens of seriously ill romusha and pleading for doctors to come at once to the camp. The ill were having seizures and contorting into bizarre postures.

The director of the hospital, Professor Tamija, then phoned Dr. Djohan, ordering him to quickly assemble a medical team to investigate what they supposed was likely to be an outbreak of meningitis at the romusha camp. Djohan worked with the adjacent Eijkman Institute often in medical research and published papers with Mochtar. He quickly phoned the institute for the assistance of two technicians trained in lumbar puncture for the diagnosis of meningitis. Djohan described disembarking from the hospital compound and meeting a Dr. Aulia (his image captured in a STOVIA photograph with Dr. Marzoeki in 1918, fig. 6) at the gates in the company of a young Japanese army physician. They both asked to join the team out of medical interest. The team hastily drove the five or so miles to the camp. This is what those first responders reported seeing upon arrival: "Arriving at Klender camp, we were surprised to find dozens of people moaning in pain; some inside houses, others lying on the ground under trees, all were contorted in unnatural postures."

These immediate clinical impressions could not be reconciled with ordinary meningitis. All of the doctors agreed in this, including the Japanese army physician. They nonetheless performed lumbar puncture on a dozen of the victims. The spinal fluid in all of them appeared clear rather than cloudy, and this steered them firmly away from the diagnosis of meningitis.

After the lumbar punctures, the three doctors huddled and shared their impressions. They thought the clinical picture, which was nearly exactly the same in all of the patients, was consistent with acute tetanus. They interviewed a camp guard and asked him about injections. The guard immediately answered positively, saying that all of the victims had been injected with a vaccine the previous week. The guard produced empty, discarded ampoules that carried the label of typhus, cholera, dysentery (TCD) vaccine manufactured at the Pasteur Institute (renamed Boeki Kenkyujo) in Bandung.

Although there were more than ninety victims on that first day, the doctors felt that they could render medical assistance only to this minority of romusha who affirmed having been injected but who had not yet developed overt symptoms of tetanus. Arrangements were made on the spot to evacuate them to the Ika Dai Gaku teaching hospital at Salemba (adjacent to the Eijkman Institute) for antitetanus therapy. Transport was arranged, and the romusha were driven to the hospital and admitted. Within a few hours, they too developed the symptoms of tetanus.

At first these romusha seemed irritable to the hospital staff, but that certainly could be assigned to seeing their friends fall into the horrifying signs of tetanus. They had watched their friends become agitated for no apparent reason. Then many of them had exhibited odd facial expressions that could only be interpreted as a smile but with nothing to smile about. Such an expression is called sardonicus in medicine, a sign of acute tetanus. Then, just a few hours later, they fell to the floor and their entire bodies arched bizarrely, their fingers and toes clutched tightly. An 1806 painting from Britain illustrates a soldier dying of tetanus and exhibiting those classical signs (fig. 25). Seeing these agonies in the ninety newly admitted men, all attending at the hospital understood that something terribly wrong had occurred at Klender.

In the teaching hospital, the admitted romusha had been consigned and confined to the same ward. Japanese soldiers stood by, not really guarding but simply watching the comings and goings of staff and the rare family members who had been notified and were within manageable distance of the hospital. The doctors had administered tetanus antitoxin serum and had reassured the patients. In less than twenty-four hours, all ninety of the admitted romusha died of the agonizing respiratory arrest by which tetanus strangles its victims.

These at least actually received the hope of therapy and reassurance from the staff at the hospital. The hundreds of others who died the same excruciating way at Klender had been much less fortunate. Not long after the ninety taken to hospital had demonstrated the classical symptoms of tetanus, the doctors phoned their contacts at Klender and asked them to immediately send everyone else still alive who had received the vaccine, along with all of the remaining empty ampoules of vaccine. The reply from Klender chilled the doctors at the hospital: the Japanese army had sealed the camp. Nothing and nobody were coming in or out.

No record exists of the events of the camp at Klender after the doctors departed with their load of ninety patients, but many hundreds were left behind and may be presumed also to have died. There is no record of anyone who was injected having survived. The numbers of dead range from the contemporary Japanese estimate of three hundred (from a Kenpeitai guard to prisoner Jatman), to the "tens of thousands" mentioned by Soekarno to his biographer, Cindy Adams. A likely number is nine hundred, the estimate suggested by Djohan, based on the numbers of ill seen at the camp and the number known to have been injected at the same time.

Dr. Bahder Djohan described a visit to the hospital by two Japanese medical professors not long after the deaths. They coaxed out of his possession the hospital records of all of the romusha patients from Klender. They politely explained that the incident should be published in a Japanese medical journal, and they wanted to study the files in order to do so. Djohan never saw the professors or the records again. Sanitation of the event was in progress.

The horror that must have been Klender in those few days in early August 1944 is difficult to imagine. Nine hundred young men twisted and agonized, much as the soldier in the painting from Britain. Visualizing the enormity of the event is difficult at this distance and, without further cues, beyond those provided by witness testimony. Perhaps the closest substitute would be to compare the event at Klender with the visually documented mass suicide and murder of the followers of Jim Jones at Jonestown, Guyana, in 1979. Klender must have looked much like the aftermath of that event, which also claimed about nine hundred lives. The Japanese faced a very big job in tidying up the Klender massacre and preserving their dignity, authority, and political goodwill in its wake.

Postmortem

Dr. Bahder Djohan requested that Dr. Soetomo Tjokronegoro, head of the anatomic pathology service at the Ika Dai Gaku hospital, take tissue from the vaccine injection site of each of the ninety dead. The specimens were sent to Achmad Mochtar for bacteriological examination. Djohan hoped that laboratory cultures would confirm the clinical diagnosis of tetanus.

Jatman, chief bacteriology technician at the Eijkman Institute working under Mochtar, received the specimens and later recounted his work and findings. His description of the lab work, provided in interview in 1970 (to Dr. Ali Hanafiah and printed in his memoir), offers seemingly contradictory statements. He described being unable to culture the tetanus bacillus from any of the injection site tissues, even though he was able to do so from another sample of the flesh of a confirmed tetanus victim (a positive control). He injected white rats with some of the tissues. "Many of them developed tetanus symptoms, but not all of them died. I could not find any tetanus bacillus in the dead rats. In the remnants of the confiscated vaccine there was also no indication of either tetanus toxin or bacillus." He did not explain how he might have been able to examine the specimens for tetanus toxin. "Looking at the results, I came to the conclusion that the cause of this poisoning was tetanus toxin." He repeats this conclusion at several junctures in his written testimony.

It may be surmised that he considered the negative findings for toxin in the ampoules as inconclusive, but the negative findings for spores and bacilli in the tissues (the rats developing signs of tetanus after being injected with those tissues) and the recovered ampoules were definitive. In other words, the absence of viable microorganisms in the ampoules, the inoculated rats, and the tissues of the victims (confirmed by positive culture from an ordinary tetanus patient), taken together with the positive findings in the rats (developing an illness like tetanus), pointed to tissues of the victims having contained tetanus toxin and apparently a lot of it, but no spores or bacilli.

The bacterial cause of tetanus is *Clostridium tetani*. It is a microbe with no tolerance of oxygen. When it encounters oxygen, it dies but leaves behind a copy of itself inside an airtight covering, a dormant spore. It emerges from that state only in an environment completely lacking in oxygen. Spores of this microbe are very common in soil almost everywhere. A typical cause of acute tetanus is a deep puncture wound that places spores of *C. tetani* into tissues lacking oxygen (typically in the spaces between bundles of muscle or dead tissue of injury). The spores awaken and the microbe begins producing a specific molecule as waste. That molecule is tetanus toxin, and it is the agent of death rather than the microbe per se.

The facts of the event in Klender speak plainly enough. The estimated nine hundred romusha came down with symptoms of tetanus almost simultaneously about a week after receiving a vaccine manufactured at the former Pasteur Institute, which was then managed by the Japanese army. There can be no doubt about vaccination as the route of introduction of tetanus toxin. Jatman's testimony of findings in the laboratory, despite his inability to ascertain toxin in the ampoules by unknown analytical methods, points to injected tetanus toxin being the cause of death in the romusha.

The weeklong pause between injections and onset of illness provides no insight on what the offending agent may have been, that is, spores, bacilli, or toxin of tetanus. The incubation period for tetanus acquired naturally, by having spores of *C. tetani* forced into deep tissue where they germinate into the toxin-producing bacillus, is typically about eight days. However, we also know from the trial of a Japanese navy captain, Nakamura, that humans injected with a lethal dose of tetanus toxin also did not show symptoms of tetanus until four to seven days later (Chapter 11).

Accepting Jatman's conclusion regarding toxin versus spores or bacilli as the offending agent, one of two possible routes of introduction into sealed vaccine ampoules must have occurred, deliberately or accidentally. The accidental route offers two possibilities: (1) tetanus somehow contaminated the manufacture of the TCD (typhoid, cholera, dysentery) vaccine (we know the ampoules were thus labeled), or (2) the vaccine was mislabeled tetanus toxoid (that technology being known at the time) and was improperly manufactured. Tetanus toxoid is an adulterated form of pure toxin that is harmless and induces antibodies that render natural toxin harmless. An error in deactivating tetanus toxin, though quite improbable, could conceivably account for such a hypothetical accident at Klender. A later chapter in this history deals with these possibilities and rejects both, leaving us the task of explaining deliberate placement of the toxin in the ampoules.

By any route or means, the vaccine manufactured by the Japanese army medical men controlling the Pasteur Institute at Bandung had killed an estimated nine hundred romusha at a highly visible model transit camp just outside Jakarta. The Japanese occupier and their nationalist friends faced a very serious challenge to the legitimacy of the romusha program and the standing of its sponsors and recruiters in the eyes of 70 million Indonesians.

NINE

Darkness

News of the deaths at Klender must have quickly reached the Japanese army high command for Java at their Jakarta HQ. We have no evidence indicating those officers had prior understanding of Japanese ownership of the event. We nonetheless consider it likely that the medical men at Bandung would have obtained their permission prior to use of the romusha as guinea pigs. In the instance of the Japanese navy men at Surabaya in January 1945, such permission was obtained, but we cannot know this with any certainty for the Klender event. Whether the high command in Jakarta understood Japanese responsibility beforehand or afterward, the men in charge would have seen the calamity for what it was: a very serious challenge to their delicate relationship with Indonesia's nationalist leaders and, in turn, to the Indonesian masses.

Those leaders had implored the delivery of young men, like the estimated nine hundred who now were corpses, into the hands of the Japanese. They did so at the behest of the Japanese occupation leaders, who were now obliged to provide political cover for the nationalist leaders against the wrath of their political base—50 million Indonesians on Java who were supposed to perceive the romusha as valued labor assets cared for by the Japanese occupier. Much depended on that carefully orchestrated deceit. Should blame for the horrific event at Klender be assigned to its actual owner, the occupier, then those Indonesians who promoted and managed the romusha program would be broadly perceived as mere dupes of a truly murderous Japanese master.

The specter of legal responsibility and possible war tribunal pros-ecution likely also weighed on the decision-making in the immediate wake of the Klender event. However, this was a more peripheral and distant issue that would probably not dominate Japanese thinking until after the more proximal political crisis had been successfully averted. Only when Allied victory loomed as more certain than in August 1944 would possible prosecution for murder begin to domi-nate their actions. We thus view the motivation for Japanese actions in this stepwise fashion: first, averting the potential political crisis and, second, protecting themselves against being held accountable for the Klender event by impending war tribunal justice.

The initially lax management of the event by the Japanese leaves little doubt that they had not anticipated the calamity. The event had taken them by genuine surprise. We cannot know if this was a prod-uct of initial ignorance of Japanese ownership of the event by the high command or their misplaced confidence that the experiment at Klender would cause no harm or attract notice.

The panicky phone call to the Ika Dai Gaku teaching hospital summoning Indonesian medical aid was likely made by Indonesian managers with the permission of shocked and frightened Japanese overseers at the camp. The access to the camp, the cooperation of the Japanese sentries to queries by the medical team, the evacuation of ninety romusha (and the physical evidence of the used ampoules) to the hospital, and the postmortem tissue samples being assiduously examined at the Eijkman Institute all indicate that at that moment, the Japanese military at the camp did not yet understand what was happening or its potentially very serious political consequences. That lack of awareness and action changed within less than a day, when the Japanese army finally sealed access to the Klender camp for sanitation. Tidying up of the ninety romusha dead at the hospi-tal would prove more difficult.

No record of the disposal of the bodies could be found, either of those in the hospital or at the Klender encampment. The romusha were a Japanese responsibility, and it is implausible they would have relegated burial to others. Sending the corpses home was out of the question, if for no other reason than the Muslim requirement for burial before the next sunset or the impracticality of such transport in tropical heat. A mass grave somewhere in the rural surroundings of Klender, if not within the camp itself, seems a reasonable supposition. So too does the Japanese army removing the corpses from the hospital for transport to such a gravesite.

The Japanese obtained (and then concealed or destroyed) those ninety treatment records under the guise of collegial collaboration between medical professionals. The Japanese obviously could not pretend the deaths had not occurred, but they could construct an exculpatory explanation. Their earliest efforts to do so may have been the sealing off of the camp in quarantine fashion, as though some dreaded contagion had taken root within the camp. Such a deceit would have been easily carried off.

However, the initial efforts at sanitizing the event seem to have missed the tissues removed from dead romusha at the hospital. The bacteriology laboratory at the Eijkman Institute worked up those specimens. The analyses described by the technician Jatman would have taken at least a week to complete, probably longer. His testimony does not mention any interruption of that work, much less seizure of the specimens. The Japanese did not seem to know the specimens were there and being processed. Given their aggressive closure of the camp at Klender—even as the last of the romusha were likely still suffering and dying—they would certainly have intervened at the Eijkman to recover the specimens had they known of them. The Japanese probably were not aware of those tissue specimens until Mochtar filed his official report of the analyses to the hospital in mid-August.

With that report, it is very likely the Eijkman Institute unwittingly cornered the Japanese on the Klender event. If it contained what Jatman described in 1970, and there is no reason to think otherwise, the report would have described the evidence pointing to tetanus toxin in the administered vaccines as having caused the deaths. Such forensic evidence very likely came as an ugly surprise to the Japanese authorities then managing the event.

From the Japanese perspective, the forensic facts, having been effectively put in the public domain, very much narrowed their options for deflection of blame. Without that Eijkman Institute report, the Japanese could have simply insisted that there had been an unfortunate disease outbreak at Klender like meningitis or a food poisoning event like botulism. The Eijkman Institute report nullified such explanations. Someone had to explain why the romusha died of tetanus en masse following vaccinations. It seems likely that Jatman's analysis, and Mochtar's honest and dutiful report of it, incited the Japanese finger of blame to point at deliberate sabotage. Such a conclusion required saboteurs—a vastly more difficult lie to construct than an ordinary disease event. But Mochtar's forensic report probably left them no choice in the matter.

Owning up to the truth of what had happened was, of course, also an option for the Japanese, but they apparently had compelling reasons not to do so. We can know with certainty that they rejected that option. The political and legal consequences of a criminal medical experiment are a plausible explanation for failing to acknowledge the truth of the event.

The facts that Mochtar submitted the report and later that he became the fabricated lead saboteur are probably unrelated. The Eijkman Institute was the only possible source of purified tetanus toxin other than the Pasteur Institute at Bandung controlled by the Japanese. Indeed, the Japanese would probably have liked to have avoided implicating Mochtar. Aside from his prominent positions, the Japanese would have had to rationalize why the alleged murderer honestly identified his own murder weapon. It is not known how they did that, but they probably reasoned that a plausible conspiracy could have taken deliberate aim at the Japanese vaccine makers at Bandung. Mochtar's report could be cited as the instrument of doing so.

Nani Kusumasudjana's unpublished 1987 memoir hints at a less subtle approach to dealing with that problem. She details an oversight of fact in Hanafiah's 1976 memoir. In the days leading up to the arrests of key Eijkman scientists, Kenpeitai investigators visited the institute and sat with Mochtar in his office. Nani wrote, "Maybe this is a misunderstanding, but at the time I grasped this: administrative people at the Eijkman reported the Kenpeitai came to the institute to ask why the results of the laboratory investigation were negative [for tetanus] while their own investigation in the military laboratory reported positive findings." Nani affirms, as do all other witnesses, that the Eijkman laboratory had and reported positive

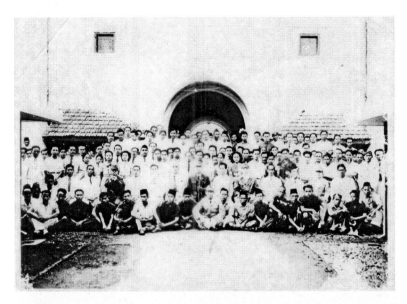

22. Staff of the Eijkman Institute, Jakarta, 1943. Mochtar is seated to the right of the Japanese officer at center. Nani Kusumasudjana stands immediately behind the Japanese officer at center right, and Ko Kiap stands behind the Japanese officer seated to the left (*to the officer's left shoulder*). Published with the permission of Nani Kusumasudjana, Jakarta.

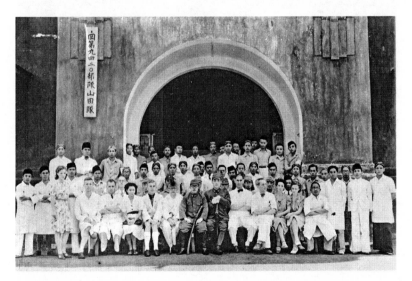

23. Staff of the Pasteur Institute, Bandung, West Java, ca. 1942. Courtesy of the Nationaal Archief, the Netherlands, NEFIS 2.10.62 inv.nr. 3036.

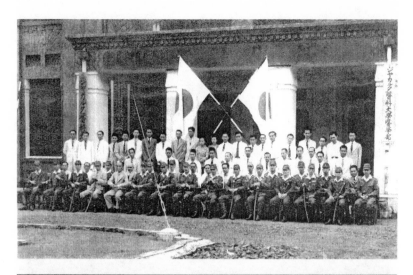

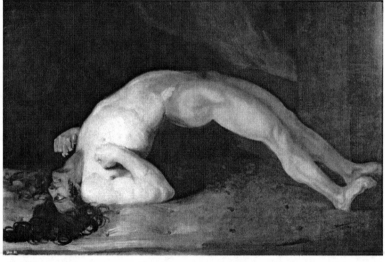

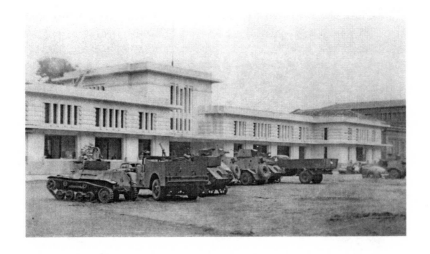

24. (*Opposite top*) Faculty of the Ika Dai Gaku school of medicine (formerly STOVIA) at the front of the Salemba campus in June 1944. Mochtar is seated fifth from the left. Published with permission of the Alumni Association of the Faculty of Medicine, University of Indonesia, Jakarta.

25. (*Opposite bottom*) *Opisthotonus* (*Tetanus*), which portrays a soldier dying of tetanus after gunshot wounds, by Sir Charles Bell, 1809. The painting is owned by the Royal College of Surgeons of Edinburgh and is published with their permission.

26. (*Above*) The Kenpeitai headquarters and jail, Jakarta, 1944. Courtesy of NIOD, inv.nr. 57296, Amsterdam.

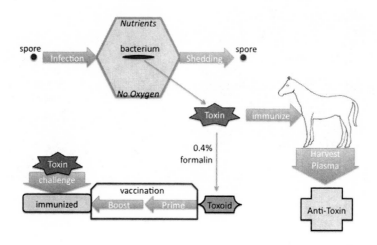

Life cycle of *Clostridium tetani*, anti-tetanus serum and tetanus toxoid vaccination

27. Diagram illustrating the production of tetanus toxoid vaccine and of tetanus antitoxin horse plasma, two distinct processes and products.

28. (*Opposite*) Poster produced by the Dutch to aid in capture of the Jakarta Kenpeitai. Courtesy of NIOD–Indische Collectie inv.nr. 481, Amsterdam.

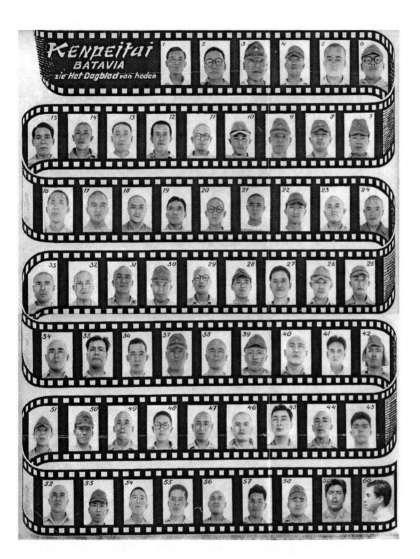

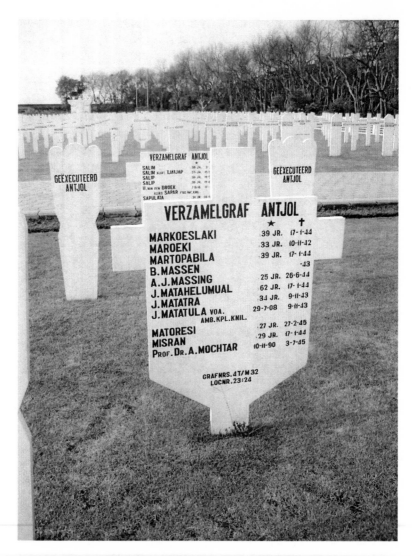

29. Placard listing Mochtar among the buried unknowns, as with the two grave markers behind the placard, which read in Dutch: "Executed at Ancol." The title of the placard reads: "Mass Grave Ancol." The edifice just visible above the horizon of tombstones at upper left is a monument marking the site of the mass grave. The site of execution is a preserved tree about thirty meters to the right of the monument. Photograph by Kevin Baird taken at Ereveld Ancol, Jakarta, in 2010.

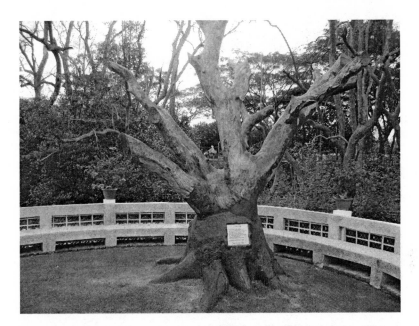

30. The tree at Ancol cemetery, reported as the site of the execution of five hundred people between 1942 and 1945, including Achmad Mochtar, on July 3, 1945. Photograph by Kevin Baird, 2010.

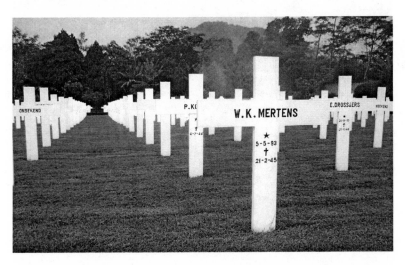

31. The grave of W. K. Mertens, the director of the Eijkman Institute in 1942, at Ereveld Cimahi, Bandung, West Java. He died of beriberi at the Cimahi internment camp. *Onbekend* on markers to the left and right is Dutch for "unknown." Photograph by Kevin Baird, 2010.

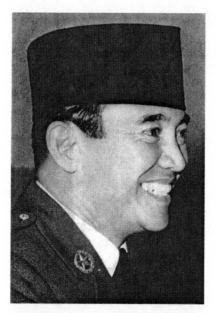

32. Soekarno in 1949. Published with the permission of the Royal Netherlands Institute of Southeast Asian and Caribbean Studies, Leiden.

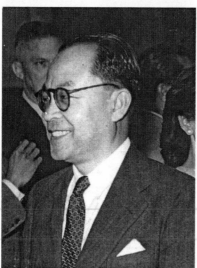

33. Mohammad Hatta in 1948. Published with the permission of the Royal Netherlands Institute of Southeast Asian and Carribean Studies, Leiden.

34. Ali Hanafiah, ca. 1965.
Published with the permission
of Taty Hanafiah D. Uzar,
Jakarta.

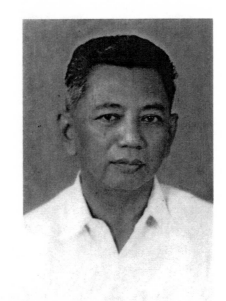

35. Marzoeki and Latifah at
Jakarta in 1947. Published with
the permission of Latifah Kodijat
Marzoeki, Jakarta.

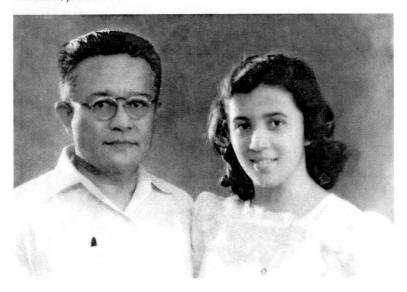

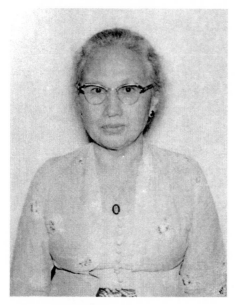

36. Siti Hasnah in Jakarta, ca. 1960. Published with the permission of Baheramsjah Mochtar, London.

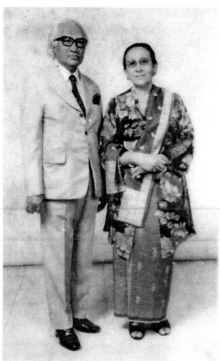

37. Abu Hanifah in Jakarta, 1977. Published with the permission of Taty Hanafiah D. Uzar, Jakarta.

38. Latifah Kodijat-Marzoeki at Jakarta, 2012. Published with the permission of Ardito M. Kodijat, Jakarta.

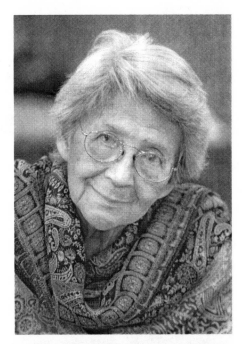

39. Nani Kusumasudjana at Bogor, West Java, in 2010. Photograph by Kevin Baird.

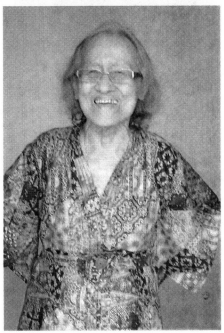

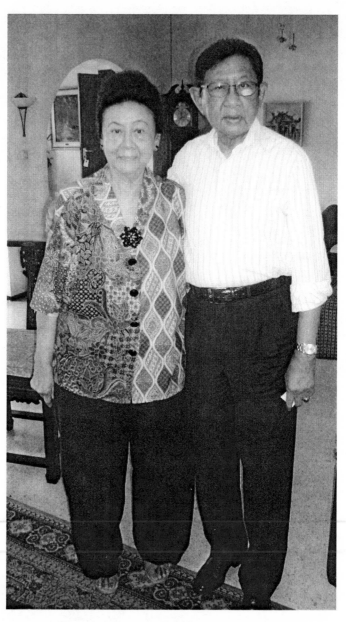

40. Taty and Asikin Hanafiah, children of Ali Hanafiah and niece and nephew of Achmad Mochtar, at Kemang, Jakarta, in 2010. Photograph by Kevin Baird.

findings. The Japanese seem, by Nani's recollection, to have mis-represented laboratory findings in order to support their framing of Mochtar for the Klender event. Another explanation may be that the Japanese perhaps referred to negative findings with respect to culturing the bacillus *C. tetani*, rather than negativity to any trace of tetanus, be it toxin or bacillus.

In any event, it was almost certainly the technical capacity to purify tetanus toxin at the Eijkman Institute that forced the Japanese—for the sake of plausibility—to construct their fabricated conspiracy upon that laboratory.

Although the romusha at Klender died in early August, nearly two months would pass before the Kenpeitai began making arrests in connection with the case. This interval likely represents time taken by the Japanese military authorities in assessing the potential fallout from their own culpability in the event and in developing solutions for its avoidance. The senior officers directly involved in managing the political relationship with the nationalists would almost certainly have been engaged in the approval and management of such a solu-tion. Too much hinged upon the outcome of this problem to leave it solely to Kenpeitai thugs.

No record of this strategic weighing is known to exist, but the long pause certainly suggests that serious deliberation occurred. Using the chain of command, where issues must reach high levels, con-sumes time. The later refusal of the leaders of the occupation gov-ernment to heed the pleas of most of the empat serangkai nationalist leadership to spare Mochtar's life points to high command under-standing of the consequences of doing so. Recall that Soekarno had already successfully pleaded to the same commanders that the life of the condemned Amir Sjarifuddin be spared. This prisoner was not only a notorious communist but also was caught red-handed as a spy in the employ of the Dutch. The stark contrast of the impo-tence of such pleas from the other three of the empat serangkai on behalf of Mochtar points to the Japanese compelling self-interests in steadfastly refusing them. In other words, it appears that Japanese military leadership had reviewed and approved the response to the dead romusha at Klender. The Japanese conspired to deflect blame to the Eijkman Institute, did so, and finally protected the conspiracy (and their own lives and liberty) by ensuring that Mochtar could never retract his confession.

Ultimately, we have only the known actions of the Japanese by which we may hope to decipher their motivation. No testimony or records relating the Mochtar affair are known to exist in the Japanese archives, be it exculpatory or incriminating. Regarding the human impact of the Japanese solution to the Klender problem, however, we have the thoroughly documented memoirs of five Indonesian survivors and the firsthand recollection of one survivor of the Mochtar affair at interview by the authors between 2010 and 2014.

Bearing Witness

Dr. Ali Hanafiah, younger brother of Mochtar's Siti Hasnah, left behind the most complete witness testimony of this event. In 1976 the Foundation for Historic Buildings in Jakarta (now defunct) published a booklet by Dr. Hanafiah, *Drama Kedokteran Terbesar* (The biggest drama in medicine). It represents not only his recollection of the events of this affair as a prisoner but also those of other victims he interviewed. Some of those accounts were extracted from scattered newspaper or magazine stories in the Indonesian press up to that time.

Dr. Hanafiah also left us a self-published autobiography that he assembled in 1977. His son and daughter, Asikin and Taty, graciously provided us with a copy of this remarkable, richly illustrated book.

Another man drawn into this tragedy was Dr. Marzoeki, who was chief of the municipal health service of Jakarta in 1944. His daughter, Latifah Kodijat Marzoeki, in 2010 provided a copy of her self-published booklet *My Parents*, written in English. This includes her parents' accounts of the events of October 1944 to August 1945 (transcribed, annotated, and translated into English by Latifah). She also provided an unedited and untranslated transcription of her father's handwritten testimony, committed to paper soon after the war. Latifah kept that original document. Her personal recollections of the Mochtar affair, communicated in interview, appear throughout this book.

Nani Kusumasudjana is the sole known surviving direct witness to the event. We interviewed her on several occasions between 2010 and 2014, and she recalled her own experience in the hands of the Kenpeitai in late 1944. She also provided us with a thirty-page unpublished memoir that she had written in 1987. Her interview and that memoir provided key insights and are cited repeatedly throughout the book.

Another important source on the Mochtar affair is the historian Theodore Friend, who until 2009 (with the publication of the *Encyclopedia of Indonesia in the Pacific War*) stood alone as the only known source on this event in the English language's historic literature. In the late 1960s, Friend became aware of the Mochtar affair (a phrase he coined) through his network of Indonesian friends, and he met with Dr. Bahder Djohan and Mohammed Hatta. The interviews of Hatta on this matter are especially important in revealing the degree to which deep concern for Mochtar affected his countrymen.

THE KNOWN VICTIMS

Before relating the events of those dark months from October 1944 to July 1945, a listing of the nineteen known victims may be useful. This is likely an incomplete listing limited to those confirmed as detained and interrogated by the Kenpeitai by witness testimony. None of the witnesses claimed or appear to have strived to provide a complete listing of the victims. Most were mentioned incidentally in the telling of their own stories.

Dr. Marah Achmad Arief: Physician in the municipal health service who administered the vaccinations at Klender. The date of his arrest is not known. He died under torture in captivity on December 9, 1944.

Dr. Suleiman Siregar: Physician in the municipal health service who also administered the vaccinations at Klender. The date of his arrest is not known. He was transferred from the Kenpeitai prison to the regular prison at Cipinang, where he died of natural causes (in the sense that no one deliberately killed him, but starvation and the lingering effects of the severe torture he endured at the hands of the Kenpeitai are certainly at blame) on May 25, 1945.

Prof. Dr. Achmad Mochtar: Director of Eijkman Institute and vice rector of the Ika Dai Gaku school of medicine (formerly STOVIA). Arrested on October 7, 1944, and executed at Ancol on July 3, 1945.

Dr. Moh. Ali Hanafiah: Physician and pharmacy investigator attached to Ika Dai Gaku teaching hospital and the Eijkman Institute. He was arrested on October 7 and released on January 19, 1945.

Dr. Djoehana Wiradikarta: Physician and scientist, he was deputy director of the Eijkman Institute and headed the serology laboratory. He was arrested on October 7 at the Eijkman Institute as he departed for the microbiology teaching laboratory at Jalan Pegangsaan in Cikini. The date of his release is not known, but he survived and briefly served as director of the institute (until being replaced by a Dutch director in 1946).

Dr. Marzoeki: Physician in charge of the municipal health service. He was arrested on October 20, 1944, and though transferred out of Kenpeitai custody in January 1945, he was not released from the city jail holding him until August 18, 1945, the day after Indonesian independence.

Mr. Jatman: Chief bacteriology technician working under the supervision of Professor Mochtar at the Eijkman Institute. He oversaw all routine work in the laboratory. Arrested on October 7 and probably released in late January 1945.

Ms. Ko Kiap Nio: Bacteriology technician at the Eijkman Institute. She was arrested on October 7, 1944, and released on November 12, 1944.

Ms. Nani Kusumasudjana: Bacteriology technician at the Eijkman Institute. She was arrested on October 14 and released on November 12, 1944.

Mr. Warsa: Bacteriology technician at the bacteriology-teaching laboratory at Jalan Pegangsaan No. 17. Arrested by the Kenpeitai on October 7, 1944, and eventually released, probably on December 23, 1944. His son, Dr. Usman, would become the chief of this laboratory and, later, rector of the University of Indonesia.

Mr. H. Mochtar: Technical assistant to Mr. Jatman, responsible for the maintenance and daily functioning of the bacteriology laboratory at the Eijkman Institute. Arrested on October 7, 1944, and released on January 19, 1945. Not related to Professor Mochtar.

Dr. Soetarman: Scientist in charge of the chemistry department at the Eijkman Institute. The date of his arrest is uncertain. He reportedly spent a week at the Kenpeitai prison and was released.

Professor Asikin Widjajakusuma: Staff doctor at the Ika Dai Gaku teaching hospital, he was mentioned only once in Dr. Bahder Djohan's testimony as having been detained by the Kenpeitai. No other details are known. He is mentioned also in the memoir of Nani Kusumasudjana, but only in the context of him being the father of her close friend.

R. Soebekti: Analyst at the Eijkman Institute, cited by the testimony of Mr. Jatman. Duration of imprisonment is unknown, but he may have been released on December 23, 1944.

Mr. Sadio: Laboratory assistant at the Eijkman Institute cited by the testimony of Mr. Jatman. Duration of imprisonment is unknown, but December 23, 1944, was his likely date of release.

Mr. Soewarto: Laboratory assistant in the serology department of the Eijkman Institute. Described by Mr. Jatman as not being imprisoned, but he was nonetheless arrested and tortured. Dates unknown.

Unknown: Mr. Jatman described the cook of the Eijkman Institute as being arrested and imprisoned by the Kenpeitai. The institute's cook is also mentioned unnamed in a *Tempo* magazine article ("The Tetanus Drama," March 29, 1975) list of the detained, along with "a few laboratory helpers."

Professor Dinger: Dutch scientist interred by the Japanese in March 1942. In December 1944 he was transferred from the Cimahi internment camp at Bandung to the Kenpeitai prison in Jakarta for questioning in the Mochtar affair. The duration of his stay and treatment there is uncertain. Dinger survived the war.

Dr. W. K. Mertens: Dutch physician and scientist, director of the Eijkman Institute until interned by the Japanese in March 1942. In December 1944 he was transferred from the Cimahi internment camp at Bandung to the Kenpeitai prison in Jakarta for questioning in the Mochtar affair. Nani Kusumasudjana's memoir affirms his presence (along with Dinger's) in a Kenpeitai prison cell near hers. The duration of his stay and treatment there is not known. He died of beriberi at Cimahi on February 21, 1945.

Nineteen people are thus known to have been detained and questioned in connection with the Mochtar affair, though this number likely excludes at least a few among the lower ranking staff members. The time and treatment in prison among the known varies between simple questioning without detention to death under torture. Most were detained for months and horrifically abused and tortured.

What follows is based on the testimony of five survivors concerning the incredible abuses visited upon these Kenpeitai prisoners: Marzoeki, Hanafiah, Kusumasudjana, Wiradikarta, and Jatman. Their testimony, given separately and committed to paper between 1948 and 1987, is almost entirely concordant. What little discordance there is mostly involves the date of Mochtar's death, cited as July 3, 13, or 18. The Dutch War Archive (Amsterdam) record of Mochtar's death, July 3, came from the Kenpeitai record of executions at Ancol.

Imprisoned by the Kenpeitai

The Jakarta Kenpeitai established their headquarters on the prominent boulevard that bordered the western edge of the vast Koningsplien (King's Square). This huge parade ground was then the center of the expanding modern Batavia (the old center being much closer to the shore). The buildings along the four edges of Koningsplien housed important colonial offices and institutions. In contemporary Jakarta, the old Koningsplien is Merdeka (Freedom) Square, with the towering Monas Monument at its center (erected by Soekarno much later). The Kenpeitai HQ on the western aspect of the square was a law school before March 1942, an irony mentioned by some of the surviving captives in the Mochtar affair. Nani Kusumasudjana remarked that she had taken a course in law at that school a few years before being taken there as a prisoner. She identified the rooms used for torture and interrogation as former classrooms. The building stands today (as do many of the colonial period palaces bordering the old Koningsplien) on Jalan Medan Merdeka Barat and is occupied by offices of the Ministry of Defense.

The Kenpeitai HQ quickly became a dreaded locale. Students in the library of the National Museum could hear from its windows the screams of victims emanating from the adjacent Kenpeitai compound (fig. 26). Several witness accounts in the Mochtar affair and other sources describe such awful screaming as having commenced when the kenpei took up residence there and not ceasing until they were evicted in August 1945. The Kenpeitai operated a torture factory: a hellish piece of real estate housing the tormented. Survivors of the Mochtar affair left us with grisly accounts of the daily functioning of that hell.

An extraordinary poster showing the faces of the Jakarta Kenpeitai survives. Returned Dutch forces produced it to aid in the capture of those men for trial after the war (fig. 28). It is a chilling gallery of the men responsible for much of the dark history relayed here.

The first person arrested in connection with the Klender event was Professor Mochtar, on Saturday, October 7, 1944. There are two accounts of his arrest. One reports him being arrested at his relocated home on Jalan Cikini Raya during lunchtime. He did not usually drive home for lunch, but on that day he had done so because Siti Hasnah had prepared his favorite dish. This seems credible. His colleagues at the Eijkman Institute appear to have had no inkling of serious trouble prior to their being collected by the Kenpeitai at the institute later that day.

These are the independent accounts of those who survived captivity at the Kenpeitai HQ in Jakarta.

DR. MARZOEKI

Dr. Marzoeki's written testimony gives the most extraordinary detail of the cruelty of his treatment at the Kenpeitai HQ. A STOVIA man and Minangkabau, Dr. Marzoeki was a senior health officer. He was working routinely at his desk in the municipal health service offices at Tanah Abang on October 20, 1944, when two Kenpeitai officers entered and demanded he come with them. He was then taken to their HQ and jail at Koningsplien. After stripping him down to his underwear, they took him to the rear of the compound where a dozen cages had been built into an area that looked like it had once been an open-air garage. The rear and only wall was brick, and the structure had a proper roof. The cages had wooden bars as thick as a man's arm. The entrance to the cage was placed a half-meter up from the ground and was only a meter tall, so prisoners had to crawl into their cages. As Marzoeki thus first entered his confinement, the guard kicked his groin and thighs.

Upon entry, Marzoeki saw half a dozen men already in the cage. In his memoir, he observed that their forlorn and broken looks gave him some sense of what the Kenpeitai had in store for him. If the prisoners spoke, the guards would strike them with poles.

After Marzoeki had languished for two silent weeks in his cage, the interrogators finally came for him. They brought him to a room within the Kenpeitai HQ building and sat him down in a chair. Without a single word being exchanged, a Kenpeitai man reared back and punched him with full force squarely on the chin. The blow knocked Marzoeki unconscious. When he came to, his interrogators simply asked for his confession, explaining that all of the others had confessed already. He did not know what it was he was expected to confess.

The questioning lasted for fifteen days. Whenever Marzoeki gave an answer that displeased his captors, one of the men would scream, "*Bohong!*" (lie) and either slap his face or strike him with a wooden, bamboo, or rubber stick. On other occasions he would be placed on an iron plate and forced to squat, enduring a wooden stick placed behind his knees and holding heavy weights for many hours. They tied his hands behind his back and then suspended him by the wrists several inches above the ground. They applied electric shocks to his genitals and elsewhere. The Kenpeitai also water-boarded him, tying him to a wooden plank, placing a cloth over his head, and putting him inclined under a fully open water tap. He underwent the sensation of drowning and lost consciousness, at which point "it was not fun anymore for them," and he was left alone to regain consciousness. Lit cigarettes were repeatedly pressed against his skin and held there, just to the point of being almost extinguished. They also would wrap paper around his limbs, one at a time, lighting it afire and watching him writhe in anguish as it burned. Marzoeki recounts all of these wretched details in his notes.

Marzoeki, at one point, asked his interrogators to simply kill him. Their reply, in broken Indonesian, was "*Tidak mau rekas rekas.*" Marzoeki, knowing the Japanese difficulty with the letter *L*, supposed that they meant to say "*lekas lekas*," or "We don't want to do that too quickly."

"The pains were so terrible that you try to forget them!" Marzoeki later reflected. "What helped, too, every time I returned to the cell I felt the sympathy of my fellow cellmates. Wasn't it strange that in spite of all the differences in religion, race, and position, during those moments friendship bonds arose? Who was not too sick or exhausted helped the newly tortured victim with comforting words, cleaning the wounds if possible or giving a massage. We felt as one, not only those within the cell but all others with the same fate."

Marzoeki was told that he would be transferred to Cipinang Prison, where he was to be shot. The date was November 12, his daughter Latifah's fifteenth birthday. (It was also the day of release for Ko Kiap Nio and Nani Kusumasudjana.) His captors instructed him to jot a farewell note to his family. The transfer to Cipinang did not materialize. The interrogations ceased on November 15.

He and others write of December 9, 1944, as an unforgettable day. In plain view of all of the inmates at Kenpeitai HQ, the body of their colleague, accomplished malaria researcher Dr. Marah Arief, showing obvious signs of severe torture, was dragged before their cages and dropped in front of them. The corpse was then wrapped and sent to his family. The message to the other inmates (and the broader STOVIA family) was clear: this can happen to you, too.

As Marzoeki later wrote, "We were in a dilemma: a forced confession to participation in mass murder meant signing a death warrant, and denial would bring torture and eventually also death."

DR. ALI HANAFIAH

The testimony of Dr. Ali Hanafiah also provides a clear picture of what happened at the Kenpeitai HQ. On October 7, 1944, he was in his office at the medical school busy preparing for his lecture in pharmacy. Mr. Soekro, the administrator at the Eijkman, found him and reported that he was urgently wanted at the institute, about three hundred meters away. He bicycled over, oblivious to what awaited him.

A Kenpeitai man in civilian dress greeted him at the tunnel

entrance to the institute. The man ordered him upstairs to the library, where he found several other Eijkman staff waiting. When he greeted his colleagues, a Kenpeitai officer at the door of the library fiercely shouted, "Shut up! Do not talk."

In short order they were transported to the Kenpeitai HQ. Like Marzoeki, he was stripped to his underwear and driven around to the back of the building, where he saw the wooden cages. He was held in cage #6, along with a dozen others. Speaking was not permitted. A soldier pacing in front of the cages would poke a long stick through the bars to strike anyone who did. A trench at the rear of the cage, serving all of the cages with a constant flow of water, was both their toilet and also their water supply for bathing.

Ko Kiap Nio from the institute, locked in an adjacent cage holding women, recognized Hanafiah and asked in a whisper if he knew the reason for their arrest. He whispered back that he did not.

Hanafiah's testimony at this point gives us some insight into not only him but perhaps also his brother-in-law, Ahmad Mochtar. In captivity, Hanafiah rediscovered his religion after long neglecting it. "I had always been occupied with all kinds of work and activities, unmindful of religious matters," he later reflected. "Only in the event of trouble did I remember Allah the Almighty and ask for His help. That was the state of my Islam when I was arrested and sent to the Kenpeitai prison."

Tellingly, Hanafiah did not describe the tortures inflicted upon him, as if unable or unwilling to revisit the memories. Instead, he wrote,

> While awaiting my fate, I had the opportunity to see and hear with my own eyes and ears, the physical torture experienced by other detainees. Screams of pain and pleas for mercy were to be heard almost every day. One morning, when Dr. Marzoeki was allowed to take a bath after he had been interrogated, I saw his back covered with red stripes and blood from being beaten with a rattan stick. From behind the bars I saw Dr. Achmad Arief, up both of his thighs were swollen and suppurating as a result of wounds he sustained during the beating. Dr. Djoehana was thrown on the grass in front of the cells, unconscious.

Darkness

A few times I saw Professor Mochtar passing my cell, his head covered with a sort of white pillow case. Although his face was covered, his manner of walking showed me how much he had suffered.

Hanafiah's memoirs relate the story of an Indonesian man visiting the home of Professor Mochtar at Jalan Cikini Raya, an incident he presumably learned of after his release. The visitor refused to give his name, but indicated that he was working for the Kenpeitai. This mysterious man may have been a sympathetic Tokkeitai officer who appears in the testimony of several others.

The Tokkeitai were the Indonesian partners to the Kenpeitai. Most of these men were veterans of the notorious Dutch intelligence agency, the Political Intelligence Agency, the PID by its Dutch initials. They were Indonesians to be feared and loathed by fellow Indonesians.

The visitor instructed Mrs. Mochtar to bring food and clothing to the Kenpeitai HQ and to use her daughters to do so. Mrs. Mochtar had no daughters to send, but she sent Hanafiah's daughter, Taty, and another two teenaged nieces, Rika and Sam, according to Hanafiah's testimony. These girls were cousins Rebecca and Nursyamsa, recalled Taty in 2013.

In a 2010 interview, Taty said of her first visit to the Kenpeitai HQ, at the age of fifteen, "I remember it vividly. We walked into the scary building's front door. Two Kenpeitai sat at a desk like a reception area. They had in front of them spread out over the entire top of the desk passport photos of dozens of women. They pointed to this one and that one, speaking in Japanese and laughing out loud."

Finally they took notice of the girls and took the parcels for Hanafiah and Mochtar. The girls would eventually visit twice more. On the third visit, the guards shouted at them, "Do not come back or we will arrest you, too!"

Hanafiah received the clothing in those parcels, but not the food. Denial of food was a weapon to which the Japanese paid scrupulous attention. When Dr. Hanafiah was released on January 19, 1945, he had lost fully one-third of his normal weight. His son Asikin recalled in a 2010 interview the day his father finally came home: "A Japanese Army truck paused in front of our house and pushed a man out of the back. The man was skinny and bald. I thought, 'Why would they dump that man in front of my house?' After a little while I realized that the man was my father."

NANI KUSUMASUDJANA

The testimony of Ms. Kusumasudjana was given at several interviews between July 2010 and January 2014 at Bogor, West Java, or in Jakarta. She is the sole surviving direct witness to events in the Eijkman Institute of late 1944 and the Kenpeitai HQ. She had considered the event a buried darkness forgotten by all involved and not broadly known. Our visit was her first opportunity to speak of the traumatic events of sixty-six years earlier.

After reading a draft manuscript of this book in late 2013, Nani contacted us and explained that she had more to report. At length, and with the strong encouragement of her son and daughter-in-law, Nani somewhat reluctantly shared a memoir of her experience that she penned and signed in late 1987. She gave us a copy, and it serves as vital documentation of what occurred in the Kenpeitai jail in Jakarta in late 1944.

After her release from the Kenpeitai prison, she refused to return to the Eijkman Institute and stepped away from science altogether. The day she was released, her captors sternly warned her not to speak of what had transpired. Even by the following year, when people asked her if Mochtar had killed all of those romusha, she could only shake her head no and refuse to speak of it. She learned of Mochtar's death much later through one of her father's acquaintances, Asikin Widja-jakusuma (one of the detainees in the Mochtar affair).

She recalled being one of the last to be arrested, on October 14. Nani attributed this to her being the youngest staffer at the institute, just twenty-three years old. But only a week had passed since the first arrests, and she lived in grim uncertainty. The Kenpeitai men indeed appeared and demanded to see her. She was with friends at a nearby restaurant when Mr. Soekro came and let her know she was wanted at the institute. "If I think back on it now, I recall that his eyes did not look directly at me. He did not have the heart for this." When she approached the institute, a young Kenpeitai man sat in the back of his sedan waiting for her. She described him asking politely in a smooth voice, "You are Nani?" When she affirmed this, he said in an almost bright manner, "Come with me." She was seated in the front of the sedan.

"What feelings came over me at the time I cannot explain. Not shocked. Maybe a little surprised. But one thing is certain: I was not frightened. That certainly sounds strange, or maybe arrogant, but that's the reality of it. Maybe this is just what people resigned to their fate feel."

After a brief stop at the nearby microbiology teaching laboratory at Jalan Pegangsaan for reasons unknown, the sedan drove directly to the Kenpeitai prison at Koningsplien. She was escorted straight away to an interrogation room. She reported not being physically abused by her interrogators, but nonetheless being shaken and terrified by their verbal ferocity. They began by explaining that all of the others had already confessed, and now it was her turn.

"Confess to what?" Nani had asked sincerely. She summarized that first interrogation like this: "Because I harbored no guilt and certainly did not understand, I answered, 'I don't know,' even though the questioning became more intense as it went on. Apparently that man's patience, which was not much, had been exhausted, and he began to make me feel guilty even though I had done nothing."

Nani was then registered as a prisoner and taken to cell #8. There she found Ko Kiap Nio and some other women prisoners she described as Eurasians. Their crime had been to produce pamphlets conveying verified news of the Pacific War.

She described what followed in the next few days:

> Every time I came back from interrogation, my confusion increased or I did not yet understand what they wanted me to confess to. They said I was an accessory with Dr. Mochtar. . . . Day after day the longer they interrogated me, the fiercer they became. I felt confused, and I was quiet when being yelled at. And when mealtime came, I had no appetite and I was not hungry. . . . After a few days of custody and interrogation, distress began to overwhelm me. . . . I faced Kenpeitai interrogators and could hear the screaming of others being tortured in another room.

She detailed one terrifying interrogation session where she felt particularly vulnerable.

One day I became desperately fearful. I was brought to a room in a house inside the Kenpeitai compound. There I was interrogated with ferocity by Kenpeitai man A, who screamed, "Confess! Confess!"

I said nothing. Nothing at all. I did not answer because I did not have an answer. After a while I could see A was becoming increasingly angry. Another Japanese suddenly barged into the room shouting that the Japanese navy had wiped out the American navy in the Pacific Ocean. He spoke in Japanese (the other man, and he always wore a white cloth hat). He repeated the news in Bahasa Indonesia. Was this news supposed to intimidate me? I thought that because they watched me for a reaction. I did not react at all. I knew with certainty their "news" was a lie.

In that interrogation in the room in the house, I saw sitting on a small table a portrait of a Japanese woman wearing a kimono. Her face was sweet. I thought maybe it was his wife or girlfriend. I studied the photo and suddenly in my heart I heard a voice say, "Speak with her." I asked her to help me survive this interrogation and get out of this house. Then I heard the interrogators say the word "electricity." They shouted at me, "We will electrocute you!" I paid no notice of them. I was talking to the Japanese lady in the portrait, a stranger. Kenpeitai A moved the portrait and forced me to look back at him. Then the two men spoke to each other briefly. I was taken back to my cell.

She continued with a wrenching description of her state of mind on that day:

When I returned to my cell, K [Ko Kiap Nio] was not there. I supposed she was being interrogated. She soon returned, her face grim, and she began screaming. I could not bear to watch. A feeling of loneliness consumed me. On the outside I looked silent and indifferent, but my own heart screamed, "God, protect me!"

At length, the Kenpeitai put before her a box of ampoules reportedly taken from the cold room in her lab at the institute, which she had entered every day as a matter of routine. She examined the ampoules and noted that they appeared, even in 1944, to be antique. The labels were handwritten in India ink and the edges appeared discolored and frayed with age. She declared she had never seen these ampoules before. She did not know what they contained.

They then questioned Nani about ampoules of vaccine kept in the cold room. She recalled that the interrogators showed a great deal of interest in these ampoules. Their origin there alleged by the Japanese interrogators seemed to represent a key piece of their argument for Mochtar's guilt, this being the only conceivable opportunity for tampering by Mochtar. But Nani could not know that. She only knew that the ampoules seemed important to them.

She controlled access to that cold room. She kept the only key. In the 2010 interview she was asked to describe the cold room. It was freezer temperature, not refrigerator. Her finger pointed to places in the cold room where ampoules of vaccine had been stored, as though she were standing in it again. Her eyes looked to the places where she pointed. She could see these things. Pointing at the floor a few feet in front of her she said, "There were glass ampoules, the ones shaped like this [making the shape of a bowling pin]. They had desiccated vaccine in them, but I did not know what kind of vaccine. There is a single box, maybe a couple dozen ampoules in it." She recalled that the box had been there since her first day of work at the Eijkman, and it had remained there up to the day of her arrest by the Kenpeitai.

Nani had understood when she was arrested that the romusha at Klender had died of tetanus. Mr. Jatman, her boss, had processed the specimens. She knew the direction of questioning was guided by an attempt to frame Mochtar, but she did not grasp her interrogators' strategy. Frustrated with her failure to corroborate their story of missing vials, they repeatedly demanded she confess. In retelling the experience, her voice rose and she fully spread her arms outward forcefully, saying loudly with fresh exasperation, "Confess to what?" Seeing her relive this horror was chilling, as though being in that interrogation room with her.

She really did not understand what it was they needed her to say. The single box of a couple dozen ampoules of vaccine in that cold room had emerged in the Japanese strategy to pin blame on Mochtar and the institute. It created the opportunity for Mochtar and others to allegedly tamper with vaccines destined for Klender. The discrepancy between the reality of their having only a couple dozen vials—versus the many hundreds that would have been required to kill nine hundred romusha in Klender—did not seem to discourage the Japanese. A whitewash is always thin in substance. The lone box in Nanny's cold room was the only piece of vaccine evidence to be found at the Eijkman, and the Japanese would relentlessly exploit its value in their concoction, no matter how pathetic its weight.

Her interrogators finally let her know what they wanted her to confess. They explained what they wanted to believe, that Nani had replaced dry culture tubes of tetanus bacterium taken by Mochtar. Her interrogator put it like this: "Nani, you played a shell game." The idiomatic expression in Indonesian (which the interrogator was speaking) for this is *tipu muslihat*. She recalled, "I looked at him with surprise because I did not understand the expression. This was because I only studied Indonesian in earnest after the Japanese arrived." She went on, "Kenpeitai man B laughed at me and explained, 'Wow, Nani always uses Dutch language, yes? Well, *tipu muslihat* means *tipu musuh lihat!*'" This is a clever play on words where the interrogator says "shell game" means "see the deception of your enemy." In her memoir, Nani added sardonically, "This is what passes for prison humor." Nani steadfastly insisted that no culture tubes or vaccine ampoules ever went missing from that cold room. She never faltered in this insistence for the simple reason of its truth.

Nani's description of the cells behind the Kenpeitai HQ was essentially the same as detailed by the men: wooden and bare. She was in the cage facing the guard post. Though she insisted her captors did not physically torture or sexually abuse her, at interview she became quiet and finally said, "They really hurt a lot of people. They treated them very badly. There was always screaming."

Nani's memoir, however, distinguishes between the Japanese guards (low-ranking regular army men) overseeing the cells and the Kenpeitai interrogators. She described her guards as not violent and even occasionally engaging in pleasant chitchat. They displayed gentlemanly respect for the women's privacy. In one remarkable episode, Nani details how the guards would conduct surprise inspections of their cells. When the shouted order came (unexpected at irregular intervals), they were required to immediately stand at attention on the spot without moving until the chief guard entered the cell to conduct his inspection. One day Ms. Ko Kiap dared to remove her shirt to conduct a quick repair. She was topless when the shout to stand at attention came, and she did so, not daring to put her shirt back on. They waited, but the guards did not appear before being stood down by another shout. The guards had realized Ko Kiap was not properly covered and elected not to enter her cell. Nani describes other kindnesses by these men, like sneaking supplements from their own meager food rations onto their stark ration plates. One guard slipped her a small bag of candies on a few occasions. They were sometimes allowed to receive the restaurant box meals dropped by their families.

Latifah Kodijat Marzoeki's reminder to not paint too broad a picture of the Japanese occupier comes to mind. Even within a Kenpeitai jail full of torture, murder, and raw suffering, one encounters the complexity of human goodness versus evil and of the events that bring those natures and choices forth. Among Japanese jailers in army uniforms, goodness and human decency prevailed for most of them. The squad of guards keeping the prisoners at the Kenpeitai jail demonstrated not only mores and relative civility but also kindness and empathy so far as their treatment of those two women prisoners were concerned. It should be pointed out, however, that these Japanese guards were regular soldiers detailed to the Kenpeitai facility. They were not inculcated into the cruel and ruthless culture of the elite Kenpeitai. The interrogators were.

Nani Kusumasudjana would spend four weeks in the jail before being released on November 12, 1944. Her memoir expresses feelings of guilt in surviving, despite having played (unwittingly), she felt at the time, a direct hand in the deaths of the romusha at Klender. She could not have then known with any certainty the fact of Mochtar's innocence, though all her deeply human instincts said so. She describes in great detail a horrific and vivid nightmare she experienced "a little while before" the end of the war, many months after her release. At the time she had no inkling that, in fact, Mochtar was either dead or soon to die, much less how. The dream seared into her memory.

Here is how she described in late 1987 the nightmare she had in July or August 1945:

And one night I had a dream. I dreamt I was on Jalan Kwitang beside the house of Dr. Asikin W. K., the father of Azil. When suddenly flashed in front of me, hundreds of empty carts just crashing down without damaging the trees or everything else that exists between the road and the road running parallel to Kwitang where I stood. The carts were just like those in a painting in which Marie Antoinette—wife of Louis XVI—stood as a prisoner on her way to the guillotine with great dignity and resignation. I'm looking at them with wonder. Suddenly I saw a man standing upright in one of the carts, among other empty carts. That man, all dressed in white, twisted his neck and looked at me. I heard his faint voice say: "I am innocent—why do you think I am guilty?" And he goes away waving from among the empty carts, still looking at me.

She declares in her memoir that it was the stirring complete recall of this dream in 1987 that prompted her to commit her memories to paper. In that year she had stumbled upon a battered copy of Hanafiah's 1976 memoir while shopping at a department store in Jakarta. She bought it and gave it a careful read. The book brought her to understand that some still doubted Mochtar's innocence. In her memoir she quotes the book (p. 27) attributing a remark to Soekarno: "The late Prof. Dr. Mochtar should have been put to death because he had killed thousands of people in Indonesia." That is when the dream bolted back into her mind, and she declared the firm belief that Mochtar had reached out to her in that dream. She felt duty-bound to record all she knew, and she did.

DR. DJOEHANA WIRADIKARTA

Dr. Djoehana's testimony is recorded as an appendix in the book of Ali Hanafiah [*Drama Kedokteran Terbesar*]. The Kenpeitai apprehended Dr. Djoehana as he left the Eijkman for the nearby microbiology teaching laboratory at Jalan Pegangsaan at Cikini. During three or four interrogation sessions they accused him of being pro-Dutch and anti-Japanese. Several times they demanded that he record every aspect of his work, documenting what it was he did on a day-to-day basis. During interrogation the Kenpeitai pushed lit cigarettes to his hands and feet, applied electric shocks, and beat him. Throughout this ordeal he insisted that the Eijkman Institute was not involved in making vaccines and that the only vaccines were made by the Pasteur Institute Bandung.

According to Dr. Djoehana, it was impossible for him to believe Mochtar to be guilty, based on Mochtar's character, his lack of opportunity to contaminate the vaccines, and the powerful motivation of the Japanese to deflect blame for the event at Klender. He also cited a similar case of tetanus vaccine deaths in Surabaya during the war (the Nakamura case described in chapter 11). This simple citation by Djoehana led us to seek and obtain a courtroom transcript of that war tribunal proceeding from the Australian National Archives.

MR. JATMAN

Mr. Jatman described much of his imprisonment, but like Hanafiah he seemed unable or unwilling to express his own experience with torture in Kenpeitai hands. He only wrote, "For days and weeks they kept interrogating me and I was constantly subjected to threats, physical abuse, and torture." Remarkably Jatman dedicated most of his testimony to deciphering Japanese intent and strategy, and in so doing he left us the most factually compelling direct testimony for grasping Japanese thinking at this time.

As Mochtar's laboratory chief, he was considered a key witness. The interrogators strived to have him corroborate Mochtar's confession of sabotaging the vaccines used at Klender.

> For many months when the investigation had slowed down, I was confronted with Prof. Mochtar for the first time. Strangely enough, in that confrontation session I was not allowed to talk to Prof. Mochtar directly. In every interrogation session his face was always covered with a cotton sack. Maybe Prof. Mochtar's face and his penetrating gaze made them reluctant to have face-to-face contact with him. I was informed that Prof. Mochtar had confessed his guilt. They claimed that Prof. Mochtar had confessed to stealing a tube of tetanus culture and had poured the contents into the bottles containing the TCD [typhus, cholera, dysentery] vaccine. The letter of confession had already been prepared and I was to sign it. I was really ignorant of the contents of that letter because it was written in Japanese charac-

ters. Because the statement contradicted the results of my examinations, I refused to cooperate. What was worse for me that if I signed that letter, I would have pushed Prof. Mochtar into his grave. Thus I entered into a lengthy discussion with the interrogators in which I claimed that the cause of the mass death was not tetanus bacilli but tetanus toxin. At great length I explained to them about tetanus bacillus, tetanus toxin, and the process of making it. Fortunately, an advisor, a Japanese doctor, was present in this discussion to confirm my explanation or, at least, to cool the heated atmosphere. I did not sign the letter.

After this, the interrogators left Jatman alone for a span of time. When they resumed questioning, it was with a document in hand which they purported to be yet another draft of the confession by Mochtar.

After Prof. Mochtar's first confession, I was interrogated again by the team. This time the Japanese doctor and Prof. Mochtar were not present. They said that Prof. Mochtar had confessed to stealing the tetanus toxin but not bacilli from the stove [incubator]. It was this toxin he put into the bottles intended for the TCD vaccine. For the second time I was instructed to sign Prof. Mochtar's letter of confession. At that moment it became clear to me that all of this had been engineered by the Japanese. Once again we got into heated arguments and I reiterated that it was not true. I did not make or store toxin. Prof. Mochtar could not possibly have made toxin by himself because the apparatus were not available in the Department of Bacteriology, especially the bacterium wax, which was stored by Mr. Soewarto in the Serology Department. . . . Possibly due to his refusal to confess he [Mr. Soewarto] was severely tortured. I stuck to my statement and refused to sign Pak Mochtar's letter of confession. I said, "If Pak Mochtar has confessed what is written here, let him sign it."[1]

Jatman, uniquely among those providing written testimony, named his tormentors. "Mr. Morimoto" is described as the interrogation team leader. We find a Sergeant Major Morimoto Arata among the faces in a poster produced by the Dutch to facilitate the capture of the Batavia Kenpeitai (he is #31 in fig. 28). He also names a Mr. Ueyama (no such

Darkness

name appears in the archival poster) as a Kenpeitai person to whom he would provide English lessons. Mr. Ueyama apologized to Jatman and admitted knowing all along that Jatman was not guilty. According to Jatman, "Upon leaving the prison he [Ueyama] said: 'Good-bye and go home safely.' I was very touched. The man who, at our first meeting had been so harsh and cruel, finally became my best friend."

Jatman also provided us with the only testimony revealing the Japanese theory of Mochtar's actions. He recalled that while in detention,

> Mr. Morimoto once told me that Prof. Mochtar was arrested because he was planning a revolt against the Japanese army. What Mr. Mochtar did was to start a germ war in Jakarta and Tangerang. His plan to do the same thing in Bogor and Bandung was thwarted. Pak Mochtar and his friends, all from Sumatra, would invade Java. Mr. Morimoto told many more stories which were intended to make us suspicious of each other.

Jatman recounted hearing a story from one of the Kenpeitai guards and a male nurse from the hospital at Tangerang. They described patients coming in with gonorrheal infections of their eyes caused by eye drops contaminated with gonococci. The doctor involved was Dr. Soeparno, formerly an assistant of Professor Dinger, a bacteriologist (and being held at Cimahi internment camp at Bandung). Soeparno was not detained, and the incident was blamed on Mochtar.

Jatman closed his testimony with a description of some investigative initiative of his own. He described tracking down Soekarmen Kertoredjo after the war. Soekarmen was the chief analyst and deputy director of the Pasteur Institute under the Japanese army director (and an Eijkman Institute alumnus). He described an investigation at the Pasteur following the event in Klender, but with no arrests being made, "because their personnel were mostly Japanese. But one of the Indonesian personnel at Pasteur informed me that a mistake had once been made in that institute. The vaccine, which was to be mixed with tetanus anatoxin [toxoid], was accidentally mixed with tetanus toxin. He said all of the vaccine had been thrown away." This testimony affirms that the Japanese in Bandung had been working on a tetanus toxoid vaccine.

On the issue of opportunity for Mochtar to perform sabotage and the alleged storage of TCD vaccines at the Eijkman Institute, Jatman's testimony does not quite square with that of his technician Nani Kusu-masudjana. He wrote, "Prior to the contamination incident, we stored a number of boxes containing typhus, cholera, dysentery vaccines in the freezer of the Eijkman Institute. These vaccines were the property of the Municipal Health Office [run by Dr. Marzoeki] and had been produced by the Pasteur Institute in Bandung. They were stored in the refrigerator to prevent them from being spoiled. People said this was the vaccine which had caused the mass death at Klender."

This key piece of testimony is frustratingly vague. Whereas Nani could point to only one box, Jatman describes "a number of boxes." He seems unable to recall the location of storage, the number of boxes, the date of their removal, or who removed them. He can cite only rumor to a possible link between those boxes at Eijkman and the event at Klender.

On almost all other counts, though, the superbly trained analytical mind of the technician Jatman gives us analytical leverage to understand this affair, much more so than does the testimony from his colleagues. Jatman asks hard questions and probes for the answers. He identifies irrationalities and indeed courageously refuses to endorse Mochtar's confession on two grounds: it would be a deadly betrayal of Mochtar, and the confession was not supported by the facts as he understood them. This he expressed.

Mr. Morimoto very clearly wanted Jatman to corroborate the conspiracy theory. His position in the lab, managing *C. tetani* cultures, would have represented a key piece of corroborating evidence. In retrospect, it is astonishing that the Kenpeitai not only permitted him to refuse the endorsement but also allowed him to survive at all. Somehow, this stubbornly truthful and rational man was spared.

The Death of Dr. Arief

The two doctors who did not survive the Kenpeitai interrogations have a unique position in this affair. Dr. Suleiman was apparently a staff physician at the Central Hospital (later Ika Dai Gaku teaching hospital) who was sometimes detailed to the municipal health service. Dr. Marah Arief worked directly for Dr. Marzoeki as a staff physician. They were the doctors at Klender who injected the romusha

Darkness

during the week before their mass death. Dr. Suleiman died on May 25, 1945, at Cipinang prison, probably of the neglect and poor hygiene at that notorious place, complicated by the abuse he suffered at the Kenpeitai prison. The death of Dr. Arief on December 9, 1944, was as a direct result of the tortures inflicted upon him. After ensuring that the other prisoners could view his mutilated body, the Kenpeitai permitted it to be sent home directly from the Kenpeitai prison. Its condition shocked and horrified all in the Jakarta medical community.

Arief's body was emaciated and completely bald (as a result of scabies, a parasitic infection of skin by mites), and his face had been beaten beyond recognition. His body bore the marks of dozens of cigarette burns. The backs of his legs had been split open from buttocks to ankles, and his family had to clean away maggots that had taken up residence in the large wounds. While all of the men had been severely tortured, none of the others met this degree of savagery, and all except Arief, Suleiman, and Mochtar survived.

It seems very likely that Dr. Arief had been made into an instrument of psychological torture for the other captives, especially Mochtar. The relative savagery of his treatment and death seems deliberate but not rationally justified in view of his peripheral role in the conjured act of sabotage. His mutilated body was paraded in front of the cages holding the other prisoners at Kenpeitai HQ. Rather than simply dispose of the body, they allowed it to go home to his family (and the community of doctors of Jakarta). Indeed, the witness testimony points to the death of Dr. Arief as an unforgettable event that deepened their already bleak, anxious state. Dr. Marzoeki recalled, "There was one unforgettable moment for us, physicians, when on December 9, 1944, at 4 p.m. we, behind bars, saw one of our colleagues, Dr. M.A., on a stretcher, dead after various tortures and maltreatment. The body was wrapped in a mat and put on a truck and sent back to the family. A wave of shock swept through the Indonesian community, but we were powerless."

Latifah Kodijat Marzoeki in 2010 recalled the day they learned of Dr. Arief's death. The news sent her mother into a fit of despair. Corrie Marzoeki summoned Mohammad Hatta to the house, and he came to console her. According to Latifah, Hatta could only say, "Cor, I understand. Trust us, we have tried everything, but we are powerless."

When the condition of Arief's body was described for Latifah during our interview, she seemed surprised and horrified. She remembered Hatta telling her mother that Arief had died because the Japanese had waited too long before seeking medical attention for his diabetes. The community had protected the families of surviving inmates from the true details of Arief's horrific death.

Nani Kusumasudjana recalled in her memoir bicycling from her home to Mochtar's a few weeks after all other prisoners had been released (approximately February 1945). She bravely did so despite her deep fear of being caught in direct defiance of Kenpeitai orders. Siti Hasnah chatted politely and mentioned that she had sent clothing in which Mochtar could pray. Nani gathered she had no idea of the severity of that prison. She recalled knowing she must say nothing about it, and wrote, "In my heart I cried out, 'Lord, do not permit her to know the real situation in that prison.'" Nani also recalled visiting the Marzoeki home while he was still imprisoned. Corrie greeted her warmly. Nani told her of when she bumped into Marzoeki at the prison and he had stolen a wink at her from behind the back of a Japanese guard. According to Nani, Corrie laughed and said, "Well, if he is winking, he must be okay."

Mochtar's Confession

All accounts of the months of October and November 1944 point to the Kenpeitai's failure to extract the confessions required for corroborating their conspiracy theory on the deaths at Klender. The death of Dr. Arief on December 9 seemingly provoked a change in Kenpeitai actions. Many prisoners were released on December 23, and almost all of them, except Mochtar (and perhaps Jatman), were released by January 19, 1945.

From Jatman's testimony we know that the Kenpeitai alleged that Mochtar had confessed to their conspiracy theory. Dr. Ali Hanafiah provided a key piece of evidence on this as well. Here is his written testimony:

> After the war was over and the Japanese troops were waiting for the arrival of the Allied Forces, upon suggestion from a friend of the family, Mr. Moh. Yamin, my two nieces, Sam and Rika, went to the Ken-

Darkness

peitai office. They were ordered [by the family] to find information in the building. They were received by a Japanese man who first refused to give them any information. But the two girls cried and refused to leave the building before they were told the whereabouts of their uncle [Mochtar]. Finally they were taken into a room, and shown a thick file of documents. Under a full-page document written in Japanese characters was the signature of Prof. Achmad Mochtar, which looked genuine [to the girls]. According to him, this was the file of the interrogation process. In this process Prof. Mochtar confessed to having contaminated the vaccines which had caused the deaths of many romusha at Klender. When asked where Prof. Mochtar was, the man answered: 'He died of illness.'

Hanafiah described the recovery of Mochtar's pocket watch (now in the hands of Mochtar's granddaughter, Jolanda van der Bom, in the Netherlands) and bloodied clothing from another office in the same building.

Sometime between December 9 and 23 Mochtar apparently signed the confession the Kenpeitai had drafted for him. Three witness accounts from that period suggest that Mochtar had made a deal with Kenpeitai, gaining the liberty of his colleagues in exchange for his signature on the confession. Hanafiah recalls an afternoon "at the end of 1944" where the prisoners were allowed to sit outside their cells, "even Prof. Mochtar, without the cover on his face. It was at that moment he had the chance to say to me: 'Please be patient, you are going to be free soon.' Those are his last words, which I will not forget. At the time I did not realize that he had said nothing about his own fate."

Mr. Jatman recalled an event on what seems to be the same day Mochtar spoke to Hanafiah:

One day a high Japanese official was to come to our prison. All prisoners were allowed to come out of their cells and sit on the grass. On that occasion I took the opportunity to talk with Prof. Mochtar and he said to me in Dutch: "They want me. I will make sure that all of you get released, but as for myself . . ." he made a gesture with his hands indicating the cutting of his throat. Once again I could not help admiring his courage and consideration for others because this meant that Prof. Mochtar would sacrifice his own life to save the lives of all of his colleagues and staff. Not long after Prof. Mochtar made his confession, all the people involved in this case were released one by one. Naturally my hopes soared but still my turn did not come and I kept on waiting."

Again, Mr. Jatman's clarity of observation and recollection gives us clear understanding.

Dr. Djoehana Wiradikarta recalled a similar experience upon encountering Mochtar in the prison toilet late in his own captivity, recalling only, "He said, 'All is fine now.'"

We know that the release of prisoners began on December 19 (although the women, Nani Kusumasudjana and Ko Kiap Nio, were both released a month earlier). These last known words of Mochtar were spoken on the day when the captives were permitted to sit together outside of their cages. This must have been a few days prior to the first release of prisoners and about a week or more after Dr. Arief's death. Mochtar's prior knowledge of the pending release of his friends, in evidence from three corroborating witnesses, could only have been obtained in discussion with the Kenpeitai, that is, in cutting a deal for their liberty. He also understood the consequences for himself, as expressed to Jatman while sitting on the grass in front of their cages. Mochtar sacrificed his life to secure the liberty of his colleagues.

Liberty or Death

Once the Kenpeitai had their confession, Mochtar's colleagues were all released. The only two prisoners who remained in custody, Dr. Suleiman and Dr. Marzoeki, were each transferred out of Kenpeitai custody and into other prisons. They were not employees of the Eijkman Institute and perhaps not included in the deal with Mochtar, or the Kenpeitai deliberately excluded them. These two men alone could provide a key piece of direct evidence exculpating Mochtar—they knew the Japanese army had supplied the vaccine ampoules used at Klender, not the municipal health service or the Eijkman Institute. In both cases the men seem to have been completely forgotten by the Kenpeitai. However, it remains possible that the Kenpeitai instructed their jailers not to permit Suleiman or Marzoeki to survive.

Dr. Suleiman died at Cipinang prison in east Jakarta on May 25, 1945. According to the testimony of Bhader Djohan to Theodore

176 *Darkness*

Friend, Slamet Imam Santoso called on Suleiman, an old colleague, at his cell at Cipinang. Santoso described him as unrecognizable, with essentially the same injuries as seen on Arief's corpse: "The Kenpeitai had tattooed him from head to toe with cigarette burns and had slashed both legs open from buttocks to heel."[2] The wounds of the still living Siregar crawled with maggots. His body was sent home to his Dutch wife. As explained by Corrie Marzoeki, Mrs. Suleiman would have had little freedom of movement to provide for her imprisoned husband. His jailers apparently made no effort at his physical recovery and possibly prohibited food from his family on Kenpeitai instructions. Dr. Marzoeki was transferred out of Kenpeitai hands, probably in January 1945, to the Tokkeitai-run PID prison directly across the street, a building that no longer exists. Latifah and her brother would bring him food every day. She recalled that a mysterious man appeared at their home one day to inform them of the transfer. He instructed them to bring food and fresh clothing. He would not identify himself, but he is perhaps the same sympathetic Tokkeitai officer who had visited the Mochtar household as well. That Tokkeitai man would have been in a position to bravely defy Kenpeitai instruction that Marzoeki not survive imprisonment. We consider him a likely explanation for Marzoeki's survival versus Suleiman's death at Cipinang prison, regardless of our speculation concerning Kenpeitai orders regarding these two prisoners.

Latifah and her brother would arrive at the PID prison around 11:00 a.m. each day. They usually sat waiting in the reception area for several hours. During this time they would hear the screams and crying of the prisoners being abused in interrogation. However, Dr. Marzoeki was not being abused at all. In fact, thanks to the relief from abuse and the food allowed and provided by his family, at the PID prison he was recovering from his Kenpeitai imprisonment. Latifah caught glimpses of him on some days and would on rare occasion even be allowed to exchange a few words as the food was handed over. Her recollection was that the Tokkeitai did not seem to understand why he was being held. They only knew he came from the Kenpeitai and, as he was Kenpeitai property, the Tokkeitai were reluctant to do anything except hold him.

His confinement lasted until the day after the declaration of independence by Indonesia on Friday, August 17, 1945, at a site commemorated in contemporary Jakarta as "Proclamation Park" at Menteng. The next day, the aforementioned Japanese civilian, Mr. Saito, phoned his congratulations on independence and earnestly advised them to go to the PID prison and demand that Dr. Marzoeki be released. Latifah and her brother Jazir dressed up in traditional Minangkabau outfits and went to the prison. They screwed up their courage and forcefully demanded that the Tokkeitai guards release their father. "The war is over. The Japanese are finished. Give him back." The guards initially dismissed them, telling them to come back after a week. The children steadfastly refused to leave and persisted in their demand. She remembered a heated discussion among several detectives. One pointed out the very real risk of retribution against the Tokkeitai by emergent Indonesian nationalists. With a shrug, they fetched Dr. Marzoeki and handed him over to his triumphant children.

They placed their father between them and walked him the kilometer or so from the prison to their home at Tanah Abang. The enormous relief of his release instantly emanated from the Marzoeki household like a joyous wave through their large community of friends and colleagues.

Marzoeki's improbable survival likely represents a Japanese error made possible by a shadowy Tokkeitai officer who bravely rendered assistance to the victims of the Mochtar affair. Marzoeki's testimony, written soon afterwards, provided one of the key pieces of direct evidence of Japanese responsibility for the deaths at Klender: they had in fact provided the vaccines that killed the romusha.

On the day of Marzoeki's release, Latifah remembers with pride, the new vice president of the Republic of Indonesia, Mohammad Hatta, appeared at the Marzoeki household to check on the well-being of his longtime friend. This was Saturday, August 18. On August 20 Dr. Marzoeki, over the sharp protests of Corrie, got dressed and prepared himself to report to his municipal health service for work. His ten months in prison became an irrelevance to him. He headed out the door, turned to his wife, and said, "We have a nation to build now."

TEN

Tetanus

The Pasteur Institute, Bandung

An injection labeled as a TCD (typhus, cholera, dysentery) vaccine manufactured by the Japanese army at the Pasteur Institute killed the romusha at Klender. There is almost no doubt that the contents of those injections included the purified toxin of *Clostridium tetani.* How this lethal material came to be in those ampoules of vaccine is the core question of the Mochtar affair. Was this done accidentally during manufacture or deliberately during or after manufacture?

Addressing these possibilities brings focus of the event at Klender to the Pasteur Institute in the city of Bandung, in the volcanic highlands of western Java. The facility was then, and remains today, the only site in Indonesia where vaccines are manufactured for use in humans.

In Dutch colonial Java, Bandung flourished as a hub attracting technical and artistic intellectuals. The Dutch referred to the city as the Paris of Java. Rich plantation owners had developed Bandung as a center of learning and as a playground that matured into an incorporated city by 1906. Nearly eight hundred meters above sea level, it offers a considerably more pleasant climate compared with steamy coastal Batavia. The intellectual influence remains in modern Bandung, home to Indonesia's vibrant pharmaceuticals industries, the prestigious Bandung Institute of Technology, along with thriving communities of avant-garde painters, writers, and musicians.

The early Dutch at Bandung were different from their relatively conservative and Eurocentric countrymen in Batavia. Planters in the

Bandung region stayed on in the colony for generations, managing the source of their wealth. With their longer and deeper exposure to Javanese culture, these planters were more likely to have surrendered, or at least retreated some, from their sense of racial supremacy. Dutch-Javanese marriages and racially mixed families of substance flourished in and around Bandung. It was a relatively progressive, tolerant, and rich city. The racist trappings inherent in a colonial existence, though certainly present, were less overpowering there.

The Pasteur Institute, erected in the northwestern sector of the city, at the edge of a quinine plantation, opened its doors in Bandung in 1895. In that era and region the Dutch were busy consolidating what would soon become a global monopoly on quinine production, then the only means of treating acute malaria. That monopoly began with a Jack-and-the-Beanstalk tale. In 1865 an English adventurer named Charles Ledger approached plantation owners in Holland with a bag of seeds for sale. Ledger's servant, Manuel Incra Manami, had collected the seeds from an isolated stand of Bolivian cinchona trees, its bark being the only source of quinine in that era. (When authorities caught Manami smuggling this precious natural resource out of the country, they beat him to death.) The stock was of extraordinary quality, producing bark containing more than five times the usual amount of quinine. The Dutch planted Ledger's specimens near Bandung, eventually driving their many competitors out of business with cheaply produced quinine. The success of the Dutch with those seeds was made possible by the decades of meticulous cinchona cultivation work by the eminent Dutch botanist Franz Wilhelm Junghuhn. He died the year before Ledger's seeds arrived.[1] By 1918 the cinchona plantations of Java produced 95 percent of the world's supply of quinine. The loss of access to that supply in 1942 sparked the development and dominance of synthetic antimalarial drugs for fifty years. Another natural compound, artemisinin from China, today dominates the therapy of acute malaria.

The early Pasteur Institute engaged in perfecting the industrial chemical extraction and purification of natural quinine. This expertise and heritage gave direct rise to the pharmaceutical industries in and around modern Bandung. The institute, however, focused most of its technical expertise and energies on the business of perfecting and producing vaccines for preventing locally important diseases. The institute thrived scientifically and productively. Vaccines against small-pox, rabies, typhus, cholera, and plague were made available there by the 1930s. The facilities at Bandung produced these vaccines in quantity, supplying much of the region before the Pacific War. The institute also developed a battery of standardized diagnostic tests widely used in the region. The Pasteur Institute at Bandung was an extraordinary asset yielding enormous health dividends all across Southeast Asia.

The building built as the Pasteur Institute today stands preserved and is occupied by a state-owned enterprise, Bio Farma. They carry on the Pasteur tradition in vaccines and produce most of the standard vaccines used in Indonesia. Jalan Pasteur is a major thoroughfare in modern Bandung. Not far from the main hospital runs a street named Jalan Doctor Otten. Otten left the Eijkman Institute to become director of the Pasteur, a post he held until the Japanese arrived in 1942. Otten and his physician scientist wife, Marie, were the institute's most prolific scientists.

Beginning in 1913 the Pasteur Institute began producing therapeutic grade antitoxin plasma for tetanus (and diphtheria). Antitoxin therapy is not a vaccine but horse plasma containing antibodies against toxin. A horse exposed to minute quantities of the toxin creates antibodies against it. Plasma from the horse, called antitoxin, is given as therapy after a likely exposure to tetanus.

Tetanus, Toxin, Antitoxin, and Toxoid

Lay writers often confuse tetanus toxin, antitoxin, and the vaccine product called tetanus toxoid. Toxoid is also called anatoxin, especially in the older literature. As has been explained, tetanus toxin is a natural by-product of the bacterium *Clostridium tetani*. This toxin, along with that for diphtheria, was discovered by the Japanese scientist Shibasabura Kitazatō (an acquaintance of both Christiaan Eijkman and Hideyo Noguchi) while working in the laboratory of the German pathologist Robert Koch.

Diphtheria is a disease caused by a bacterium that produces a toxin similar to tetanus. In both diseases the toxin is largely responsible for the catastrophic consequences of infection from the bacterium producing it. In the 1880s, once these toxins were known, other scientists immediately raised therapeutic antibodies for diphtheria and tetanus in horses. These were lifesaving advances in medicine.

However, the antitoxin plasmas are imperfect and risky therapies. They carry a number of inherent hazards. Among them is contamination with the toxin itself. The horses used to produce the antibodies could become naturally infected with the bacterium without showing overt signs of disease (thanks to their antibodies) and could contaminate the plasma with toxin. Such an accident in Texas in 1919 killed ten children and sparked the birth of what is today known as the U.S. Food and Drug Administration.

The invention of tetanus toxoid made antitoxin plasma virtually obsolete by effectively preventing the disease. Tetanus toxoid is toxin that has been treated with formaldehyde. This chemical treatment, properly done (and easily so), robs the toxin of its ability to cause harm but does not diminish the ability of the immune system to generate antibodies that can effectively neutralize natural toxin. Gaston Ramon and Christian Zoeller at the Pasteur Institute in Paris worked out this neat trick for diphtheria in 1924. Their colleague P. Descombey achieved it for tetanus in the same year.

This new technology was not easily translated to industrial scale, and it would not find broad application for ten to twenty years. It is the same technology that produces today's vaccine against tetanus, and over the decades several billion doses of tetanus toxoid vaccine have been produced. The relative rarity of that dreaded disease today, along with diphtheria (once a major killer of children), is thanks to the toxoid technology discovered by Ramon, Zoeller, and Descombey at the Pasteur Institute of Paris.

Tetanus toxoid suffers no patent rights, and over the decades the vaccine has come from dozens of production facilities representing a wide range of technical sophistication. Nonetheless, apart from the possibility represented by the incident at Klender, throughout the history of tetanus toxoid technology absolutely no deaths resulting from tetanus as a consequence of faulty vaccine manufacture are known to have occurred. The Texas deaths due to tetanus in 1919 were by horse antitoxin plasma, a wholly different product and technology.

According to written testimony from several involved in the Mochtar affair, Dutch scientists at the Pasteur Institute in Bandung had been experimenting with production of a single vaccine preparation against TCD and tetanus. They had been ordered to add tetanus toxoid to this mixture by the Dutch military authorities (KNIL) in preparation for the combat anticipated in the defense of Java against the Japanese. In a civilian public health sense, tetanus was a minor problem causing relatively few deaths compared with the heavily endemic infections the scientists typically focused their energies on. However, tetanus in that era represented a very serious threat to any wounded soldier. It was an important problem of military medicine. As the threat of war and combat loomed closer, the Dutch acted to get access to tetanus vaccination.

The experiments conducted at the Pasteur Institute in Bandung, according to Hanafiah and Jatman, suggested that safety tests in laboratory macaques proved unsatisfactory. According to accounts relayed to them, all of the monkeys died when vaccinated. The initial runs of vaccine produced there seemed faulty. Jatman describes that production run of tetanus toxoid vaccine (TCD + tetanus) being set aside for proper disposal. He speculates that the Japanese may have seized control of the institute before the vaccine could be destroyed, implying further that those faulty vaccines could have been injected into the romusha. This testimony is likely the genesis of the widely held belief within the Indonesian medical community that the Klender event was a consequence of industrial accident.

Just as the Dutch had been before them, the Japanese began contemplating protracted warfare in Indonesian jungles and paddies as it became clearer that their war fortunes were going very poorly (sometime in early 1944 seems likely). They became keenly interested in protecting their troops against tetanus, which would have been a deadly adversary in the sort of combat they had in mind. The Japanese army high command on Java undoubtedly would have given priority to the development and testing of a suitable tetanus vaccine. They now owned and operated the Pasteur Institute facilities in Bandung and, therefore, certainly had the capacity to do so.

The accounts of Hanafiah and Jatman of the flawed vaccine produced by the Dutch are both secondhand. Neither had involvement
in nor access to the results of the safety evaluation of the reported
initial TCD + tetanus product. It remains possible that the macaques
died not as a result of vaccination with a contaminated vaccine but
as a consequence of normal safety testing or in evaluating protective
efficacy. However, the Dutch scientists at Pasteur very likely would
have tested the safety and efficacy of their new tetanus toxoid vaccine in guinea pigs before exposing the more expensive macaques.
It is virtually certain that both models were employed before advancing to an industrial-scale production run for tens of thousands of
KNIL soldiers.

The published medical literature from the institute at Bandung
during the 1930s lets us know that they routinely used both guinea
pigs and macaques to test vaccines in this manner. Those records do
not include tetanus toxoid vaccine per se, simply because they had
not yet undertaken that task. That would come only as the Japanese
armed forces veered toward them.

The testing of the safety and immunogenicity of a tetanus toxoid vaccine would have been done first in guinea pigs and then, just
prior to manufacture for human use, in macaques. In both animal
models the evaluation would have been a simple matter of prime
(first exposure to the antigenic material, toxoid, in the vaccine) and
then a boost (the second shot with the same material, which provokes
a much more vigorous antibody response than the primary shot).

The scientists would then look for the ideal amount of toxoid
(dose) and interval of dosing, and use the levels of specific antibodies achieved as their yardstick for technical success. When they were
satisfied they had optimized the formulation and delivery schedule
of the vaccine, they would then move on to evaluating how well it
prevents acute tetanus in laboratory animals challenged with natural unadulterated toxin.

The evaluation of the protective efficacy of a tetanus vaccine involves
injecting ordinarily lethal doses of purified tetanus toxin into immunized animals. Scientists can measure how well the vaccine works

by first seeing that immunized animals survive the challenge with toxin and then seeing how much the dose of toxin must be increased to overcome that protection and kill the experimental animal. For example, dose x of toxin normally kills an unimmunized animal, but a dose of $500x$ is required to kill immunized animals. This gives a clear idea of the degree of protection afforded by the vaccine and therefore its protective quality.

In this light, we can see that even with a completely safe and effective vaccine, some animals in the laboratory will be killed during the normal course of its development and validation. So we cannot reliably assert that what Hanafiah and Jatman heard from Pasteur Institute workers was actually the production of a vaccine that killed animals during attempts to immunize them. Nonetheless, we may reasonably accept that the KNIL asked the Pasteur to take up the production of tetanus toxoid for vaccination of troops, and that institute tried to do this with its TCD product relatively soon before the arrival of the Japanese.

The Dutch at Bandung would be producing tetanus toxin, both for its conversion to harmless toxoid vaccine material and unadulterated and purified toxin for use in evaluating vaccine protective efficacy. The institute had certainly been producing purified tetanus toxin for use in generating antitetanus plasma from horses for decades. When the Japanese arrived, they would have found a well-developed capacity for tetanus toxin production. They may also have discovered Dutch plans and perhaps data on producing tetanus toxoid vaccine as an adjunct to the standard TCD formulation.

Boeki Kenkyujo, 1942

When the Japanese took control of the Pasteur Institute in early 1942, they renamed it the Boeki Kenkyujo. A photograph shows the staff posed at the main entrance with a banner carrying its new name (fig. 23). The photo is not dated, but it must have been not long after the Japanese arrived. The Dutch staff scientists appear in the photo, each of them pensive and uncomfortably posed. The new directors in the uniform of the Imperial Japanese Army (complete with samurai swords) are seated front center. The man in the bowtie seated on the left of the Japanese officer is Professor Lou Otten, at this time the immediate former director of the institute. He had won lasting fame on the Dutch soccer team at the 1908 Summer Olympics. His stature and bearing in the photograph suggest such. His successor was Lt. Gen. Dr. Matsuura Mitsunobu. He does not appear in the photograph, probably taken prior to his arrival, but his photograph does appear in a local newspaper editorial in 1943.[2]

Otten developed the dry, heat-stable formulation of smallpox vaccine production that, decades later, played a significant role in the eradication of smallpox as a disease. His wife, Marie, had died in 1940, and she pioneered rabies vaccination technology. The Pasteur staff conducted the basic science and very hard work that generated the local production of vaccines for cholera, typhoid, typhus, rabies, plague, and smallpox.

Otten survived captivity but died at The Hague in November 1946, just weeks after his repatriation. The image of this dedicated and great man of science and medicine in front of the institute he was instrumental in building, flanked by men bearing swords, in many ways captures the spirit of the Japanese occupation of Indonesia. The Japanese would tap the talents of the Dutch scientists for a brief period and then discard them to the nearby Cimahi internment camp. We don't know how many survived the starvation and neglect imposed upon them in that captivity.

Ankje Zuidema discovered documentation of Japanese management of the Pasteur Institute among Indonesian newspapers archived at the Nederlands Instituut voor Oorlogsdocumentatie (NIOD) in Amsterdam.[3] Japanese propagandists broadcast the institute as a center of vaccine production. The prominent Japanese serologist K. Kurauchi bragged that the Boeki Kenkyujo would supply vaccines for all of the southern Japanese Empire. This was not a hollow promise. As the newspapers explain, the staff of the institute increased from a few dozen to several hundred by late 1944. Classifieds from Bandung newspapers at that time carried ads recruiting technicians to work at Boeki Kenkyujo. The Japanese were seriously ramping up the facility.

The Japanese would surely have been reluctant to attribute the calamity at Klender to the Japanese scientists at their highly touted and strategically important production facility. It would have been seen as an unacceptable admission not only of gross incompetence and fallibility but also of the risks inherent in accepting any of their many products. This view could readily account for an elaborate and murderous cover-up in the wake of the catastrophe at Klender. But the plausibility of this theory, of course, hinges upon the romusha deaths actually being an accident of poor manufacture.

We are left to wonder how the Japanese investigated the event at Klender in order to satisfy themselves, internally at least, that such a horrific event that risked their credibility and success would not occur again and that any future production flaws, if they occurred, were quickly discovered and corrected. The Japanese almost certainly conducted an honest investigation for themselves before deciding upon espionage as the cause to be purveyed for public consumption. However, no such records have been discovered. We know that the incident in Klender occurred in late July and early August of 1944 and that arrests in connection with the deaths started on October 7, 1944. The Kenpeitai would certainly have managed the investigation rather than the Japanese army medical men in Jakarta. Those at the institute in Bandung almost certainly would not be given investigative responsibility. Indeed the Japanese medical officers at Bandung would have also faced intense and perhaps even abusive grilling by the Kenpeitai. That would have been the case had the experiment been carried out without prior approval from command. Soekarmen Kertoredjo, deputy director of the Pasteur Institute, reported no arrests being made in connection with the investigation there, citing the fact that Japanese scientists almost wholly dominated at the Boeki Kenkyujo. Nonetheless, the real truth of the fatal intoxications at Klender—flawed production at Bandung being just one possibility—probably emerged fairly quickly and informed Japanese decision-making in managing the aftermath of the event at Klender.

What we know with certainty about the involvement of the Pasteur Institute/Boeki Kenkyujo can be summarized as follows:

The Pasteur Institute had been safely producing tetanus antitoxin serum for therapy of tetanus exposure since 1913, and this involves expertise in producing and managing purified tetanus toxin.

Tetanus toxoid vaccine production was a relatively new technology in 1942, and there is no evidence of the Pasteur Institute producing it successfully before being ordered to do so by the Dutch military authorities on Java soon before occupation.

The Japanese arrived in Bandung before the industrial production of tetanus toxoid vaccine had been achieved.

The Japanese took direct and complete control of the institute.

The Japanese touted their facility as proof not only of their goodwill toward the Indonesian people but also of their technical prowess.

The Japanese at Bandung produced the vaccine injected into the romusha at Klender, and it had not been in the custody of Indonesian doctors prior to its use.

The Accident Hypothesis

Most published accounts of the Klender event blame flawed vaccine production for the romusha deaths. No direct evidence supports this explanation, and it has never been presented with a technical examination of the process of tetanus vaccine production. The vaguest notions have been inferred of the bacterium, its spores, or natural toxin somehow contaminating the production process. The plausibility of such an accident has, up to now, not been critically assessed on the weight of well-known and verifiable technical facts.

Both the biology of *Clostridium tetani* and the most basic procedures in the preparation of tetanus toxoid, along with the institute's decades of experience with sophisticated vaccine production at Bandung, leave almost no possibility that the event at Klender occurred by industrial accident. What follows here is a consideration of the technical facts supporting that conclusion.

A paper published in the *American Journal of Public Health* in January 1943, reflecting the publicly available technology of the day, details the preparation of tetanus toxoid vaccine for use in U.S. troops.[4] The starting material is bacteriological broth in flasks growing *C. tetani*, which excretes the toxin. An important fact about *C. tetani* is its identity as an obligate anaerobic bacterium. That is tech-speak for the fact that the microbe has no tolerance whatsoever for oxygen—it is as poisonous to the bacterium as cyanide is to us. If an evil person poured a test tube full of these bacilli into your milk, the exposure to normal oxygen levels in the atmosphere (and your milk) would kill the bacilli. The intestinal tract does not offer an environment free of oxygen, and the spores of *C. tetani* would pass harmlessly through it.

Under the microscope, the living bacilli of *C. tetani* resemble little tennis rackets. The head is the internally held spore. Once exposed to oxygen, the bacillus dies and the spore remains. The spore buds only when it finds itself in an environment completely lacking in oxygen. And this is how cultures of *C. tetani* must be coaxed into growth and production of toxin—by providing an environment void of oxygen. A vaccine production line would not offer any such opportunity at growth beyond the obvious first step of growing the bacillus in a necessarily and deliberately created oxygen-free environment. Such an environment is not a trivial task, and it is highly improbable it could be achieved by happenstance and with catastrophic consequences.

The broth used to grow up *C. tetani* and harvest its toxin would be rich in the bacilli. After the necessary and inevitable exposure to oxygen, the dead bacilli would leave behind their spores. The viable spores would certainly pose a hazard if injected into tissue. However, filtration techniques used in the 1940s were more than sufficient to deal with this risk. The broth would be filtered to remove the spores and much else in the messy broth. If the filtration had been somehow inadequate and spores escaped into the filtrate, this contamination would become obvious during the preliminary testing of the filtrate in animals to determine the amount of toxin present.

According to U.S. government standards of 1943 (cited by Long), the broth harboring live *C. tetani* (until exposed to air) must possess a toxin potency of at least 10,000 guinea pig minimal lethal doses (MLD) per milliliter. In other words, a few drops of broth contain enough toxin to kill ten thousand guinea pigs. This is measured by exposing guinea pigs to dilutions of the broth—all concentrations stronger than a 1:10,000 dilution must kill the guinea pig. Once toxin potency and concentration has been established, formaldehyde is added to the broth to a final concentration of 0.4 percent and, after being refrigerated twelve hours, the broth is again filtered. The toxoid so produced is then tested for complete inactivation to toxoid by injecting a whopping 5mL into a single guinea pig. That is, the animal is exposed to a dose of toxin/toxoid that is at least 50,000 times in excess of a lethal dose. The animal must remain healthy for the solution to be considered safe for use, having safely converted to tetanus toxoid. Obviously, any spores in that 5mL injection would result in death of the test animal and the flawed filtrate being discarded.

A tetanus toxoid solution that did not kill the experimental animal is then evaluated for its immunogenic character (amount of antibodies produced) and protective efficacy of that against natural tetanus toxin. One milliliter of the solution is injected into another guinea pig. When that animal proves protected against a challenge with tetanus toxin at a dose ten times the minimum lethal dose, the solution is considered adequate for toxoid vaccine production. This fact is key—challenge with purified natural toxin with survival of the vaccinated test animal proves that the toxoid vaccination actually works. We believe this lone fact represents the kernel at the core of the Mochtar affair.

A responsible and experienced laboratory, such as the Pasteur Institute, would have carried out these relatively simple and inexpensive tests using not single animals but batches per treatment group. And the better labs would evaluate in monkeys before advancing to vaccine production for use in humans. We know the Pasteur Institute used both animal models. Certainly the supply of macaques, which occur in natural abundance on Java, would have been relatively inexpensive and limitless.

We know guinea pig tests were carried out at the improvised Japanese navy laboratory at Surabaya in their production of safe tetanus toxoid vaccine. It is implausible that the far more seasoned and sophisticated vaccine production factory and laboratory at Bandung would have failed to undertake at least a similar and probably a far more thorough testing in preparing a toxoid vaccine for industrial production. The notion of live bacilli or active toxin somehow "slipping through" toxoid production and killing people at the receiving end of routinely produced vaccine was virtually impossible, even in 1944.

Finally, an examination of the chemistry of tetanus vaccine provides further doubt about the possible accidental killing of the romusha by a faulty production run of tetanus toxoid. The concentration of tetanus toxin in any given sample is not directly measured. It is historically measured by the easiest means available, that is, by the amount that could kill a single guinea pig, or the minimum lethal dose (MLD). Thus a solution that contains 1,000 MLD holds enough toxin to kill one thousand guinea pigs (or, more practically and humanely, if we dilute it less than 1,000-fold, it still kills a single guinea pig).

A key question in the Mochtar affair is how many MLD of toxin converted to toxoid would be included in a routine vaccination against tetanus? In other words, if the detoxification of tetanus toxin had been somehow completely overlooked, much less being less than 100 percent efficient in converting toxin to toxoid, would it kill a man? The answer is almost unequivocally no.

A standard tetanus vaccine is 0.5mL of a solution containing five flocculation units of toxoid. The flocculation unit was invented to create a handier and more humane way of measuring toxin than killing a bunch of guinea pigs. A 1958 research paper demonstrates the mathematical correlation between MLD and flocculation units. In that work A. J. Fulthorpe showed that 0.87 flocculation units was chemically equivalent to 0.01 MLD units. Therefore, the five flocculation units contained in a single 0.5mL standard tetanus toxoid vaccination are equivalent to 0.05 MLD units. In other words, a human being given a standard tetanus toxoid vaccination receives only one-twentieth the amount of toxin (converted to toxoid) sufficient to kill a guinea pig. The complete failure to convert toxin to toxoid would be very unlikely to kill a man.[5]

A review of the facts of tetanus toxoid vaccine production and vaccination leaves almost no possibility that the romusha at Klender had been killed by benign technical incompetence. First, there is no known precedent or antecedent industrial accident with tetanus toxoid vaccination. The simplicity and certainty of safety assessment explains this fact. Also, the dose of toxoid put into humans represents only 5 percent of the amount of toxin (converted to toxoid) required to kill even a guinea pig. The probability of a vaccine production run being so egregiously flawed that it kills 100 percent of nine hundred injected romusha must be considered so unlikely that it must be dismissed as a possibility.

This dismissal forces us to turn to the other possible explanation: that the toxin that killed the romusha at Klender had been put deliberately into the ampoules and had been in amounts of toxin far in excess of toxoid administered in ordinary vaccination. The operative question becomes: Who put it there and why?

The Kenpeitai would have us believe that Professor Mochtar and his co-saboteurs at the Eijkman Institute used cultures of *C. tetani* to adulterate the vaccines used at Klender. We have already examined the single piece of evidence in support of their theory: Mochtar's confession to doing so. We also saw from Jatman's testimony that when he explained how it was impossible for tetanus bacilli to have caused the calamity at Klender, the Kenpeitai went back to Mochtar and had him sign a new confession (using toxin rather than bacilli) consistent with this new understanding of the technical facts. Jatman then explained to the Kenpeitai how toxin production in Mochtar's lab at the Eijkman was also impossible, a clarification and understanding that sent the Kenpeitai back to their torture drawing board—having the man at Eijkman (who managed toxin purification materials) confess to producing the toxin for Mochtar in order to buttress yet another draft of the confession with technical consistency. Mochtar appears to have been confessing to whatever the Kenpeitai put in front of him. The truth had long ceased to matter to either Mochtar or the Kenpeitai.

In rejecting Mochtar's guilt and the possibility of industrial accident, we must address the question of Japanese motivation for deliberately putting tetanus toxin into a vaccine administered to hundreds of romusha. Why would they do so? Testimony in a parallel incident, from Japanese naval officers tried for the murder of fifteen condemned Indonesian prisoners at Surabaya in East Java in early 1945, sheds critical light on this question. Its examination reveals the compelling technical and military strategic reasons for exposing humans to natural tetanus toxin, along with a demonstration of the willingness of Japanese military medical men to readily overcome the abhorrent ethics of doing precisely that.

ELEVEN

Modus Operandi

Jakarta, 1945: Crime and Punishment

After the Japanese surrender on August 15, 1945, the Java Kenpeitai largely obeyed their final orders from Tokyo to aid in maintaining law and order until the Allies arrived to take over. Indonesian republican irregulars seeking weapons—they had not yet taken the shape of a national army—attacked scattered Kenpeitai barracks at Surakarta, Surabaya, Madiun, Semarang, and Bandung. The Japanese manning those barracks resisted, and many dozens of kenpei were killed. After British armed forces arrived in Jakarta and Bandung in September, some kenpei there tried to flee into the Java countryside and melt into the local population. Instead, mobs discovered and promptly killed most of them. In an odd and stark contrast, the Kenpeitai on Sumatra (under a different army command) apparently joined the Indonesian rebels in substantial numbers and gladly shared whatever weapons they had. Their ultimate fates are unclear.

The survivors of the ravages of vigilantes on Java were arrested, imprisoned, and tried by the Dutch military authorities at the Temporary Tribunal in Batavia (the Dutch still referred to Jakarta by that name) beginning in August 1946. Most of the Java kenpei who were tried in Jakarta received lengthy prison sentences, but more than thirty were executed. The commander of the Jakarta Kenpeitai, the boyish-looking Cho Konosuke (he is #60 in the poster of Jakarta kenpei) was executed at Glodok Prison on December 30, 1947. Murase Mitsuo (his photo does not appear in the poster) headed the Tokko division and was considered the mastermind of the brutish Java Kenpeitai kikosako tactics. He was executed at Jakarta on November 3, 1949, at the age of forty.[1] None of the executions were connected to actions in the Mochtar affair.

The records of the Temporary Tribunal show Kenpeitai officers convicted of mistreating prisoners in connection with the Mochtar affair. However, there is no mention of anyone being held to account for the death of Dr. Arief, the execution of Mochtar, or the hundreds of dead romusha at Klender. It may be that Allied legal officers examined the case and expediently took Mochtar's forced confession at face value. It is not difficult to imagine legal triage taking place at that time, with wholesale culling of any charges that did not look like slam-dunk convictions. Those alone kept the legal teams busy for a decade.

In Mochtar's case, the execution of an agent allegedly in league with one's declared enemy in wartime is not a crime, provided a legal process is followed. Mochtar had formally confessed that this was exactly what he represented—an enemy saboteur who had murdered hundreds of people working on behalf of the empire of Japan. His file, if it was examined, may have attracted no more than a quick read and a toss into the "too hard to do" box.

We are left to conclude that the tribunal prosecutors made no formal examination of the accusation aimed at Mochtar. In their preliminary examination, they would see that Mochtar admitted to contaminating the vaccine given to the romusha. That confession file (likely the same one seen by Sam and Rika, Hanafiah's nieces) was probably delivered intact and cleansed of any references to torture, and it officially sealed the case of the dead romusha at Klender. This single action vindicated, in a legal sense, Japanese management of the entire Klender problem. They got off scot-free.

This was also true of their political crisis with the Indonesian nationalists in the immediate wake of the event at Klender. The Japanese military occupation government, the Gunseikanbu, clearly understood Mochtar's stature in the Indonesian community and the amount of goodwill that executing him would cost. They thoughtfully called in the Indonesian political leaders and carefully laid out the Kenpeitai-constructed case against Mochtar. Heedless of their own political risk in doing so, most of these leaders repeatedly petitioned the Japanese to spare Mochtar's life. According to Hatta in 1968, he gathered Mansyoer, Dewantoro, and Oto Iskandar di Nata. Absent Soekarno, this was the empat serangkai top of nationalist leadership (excepting Iskandar di Nata, who was nonetheless a powerful politician).[2] They obtained an audience with Adm. Yamamoto Moichiro, chief of staff of the Gunseikanbu and, at least in principle, the head of state. The Indonesians pleaded earnestly and directly to Yamamoto for clemency for Mochtar. He dismissed them, weakly explaining that the Kenpeitai fell outside his chain of command.

Theodore Friend writes of the failure to save Mochtar:

> In the nine months [actually it was eleven] between the romusha deaths and Muchtar's [sic] execution, why did Sukarno not intercede on the doctor's behalf? . . . One may infer that he dreaded the Kenpeitai and readily found reasons not to cross them.
>
> As for Yamamoto, there is no evidence of his being willing to alienate the Kenpeitai, no matter how elevated his rank, on any crucial matter. Agencies of repression have a way of intimidating everyone, not just the obvious targets. Men who have the power to disapprove prefer to be too busy to oppose, and become inert accomplices. Indonesians, Filipinos, and other Asians, however, found little solace in the fact that Japanese regular army personnel feared the Kenpeitai as much as they.[3]

By this general explanation of the failure to win clemency for Mochtar, reprieve for any condemned prisoner of the Kenpeitai would seem improbable or impossible. The clemency granted to Amir Sjarifuddin, the communist and spy reporting to the Dutch, tends to dispel that notion. Another interpretation—in light of Amir's case, and the many other reprieves granted to condemned Indonesians at the behest of nationalist leaders—is that Yamamoto grasped the looming legal consequences that would result if Mochtar were ever permitted to retract his coerced confession. Mochtar surviving the occupation to tell his side of the story to the Allied authorities would certainly have provoked an exploration of who actually killed those romusha at Klender. Yamamoto likely acted to protect himself and other Japanese military men from impending war tribunal justice by ensuring that Mochtar's execution was carried out. Indeed, as explained below, Yamamoto would have received orders from Tokyo to dispose of any evidence considered supportive of war tribunal prosecution.

The Japanese seem to have hesitated in carrying out the sentence. Seven long months would pass between his confession and execution. They appear to have been watching and weighing their risk of exposure to war tribunal justice, which elevated with each passing day in early 1945. Their Nazi friends submitted to unconditional surrender in early May. The wretched and hopeless defense of Okinawa began in April and, after enormous loss of life and materiel, drew to Japanese defeat by mid-June. Her once mighty naval fleets and air armadas were now ghosts. Most of Japan's cities and industrial centers lay in utter ruin. War tribunals were already in progress in the liberated Philippines. When Mochtar's captors decided that an unconditional surrender to the Allies was inevitable, they murdered him. What the Indonesians thought of their loss had become irrelevant. Mollifying the nationalists—or anyone else but the looming war crimes tribunals—had become pointless for the men who had managed the occupation forces and now faced certain accountability for their actions.

Beginning in late 1942, the U.S. government communicated protests to the government of Japan (through the Swiss embassy in Tokyo) containing evidence it had gathered of war crimes committed by the Imperial armed forces. These protests continued throughout the war. In mid-1944, when the Japanese military began to worry about actually being held to account, they began ordering the destruction of evidence considered supportive of charges of war crimes.[4] In the few days leading up to the August 15, 1945, surrender, Imperial military command in Tokyo dispatched encrypted instructions throughout the Pacific ordering the destruction of all evidence.[5] In carrying out his execution, Mochtar's captors acted in accordance with the mien and directives of Japanese command with regard to minimizing their exposure to criminal justice proceedings.

In consideration of this context, let us drive the last nail in the coffin of the industrial accident hypothesis in the event at Klender. Recall that the impetus for framing Mochtar in such a scenario could only have been to avoid the perception of incompetence in their med-

Modus Operandi

ical men at the vaccine production facility at Bandung. Such a perception would harm their carefully guarded image as infallible and superior, as well as the vaunted success of their substantial investments in vaccine production at the Boeki Kenkyujo. These concerns would certainly evaporate with impending military defeat and consequent lack of prospects for a future in Indonesia.

Further still, had the deaths of the romusha been a manufacturing accident, it would not be a source of severe legal anxiety to the soon-to-be-vanquished Japanese army. Accidents happen, sometimes very bad ones. People are held to account only if gross negligence or criminal incompetence plays a significant role. Someone might actually go to prison, but not for very long. While such a prospect might upset ordinary law-abiding citizens, the Japanese occupiers were by no means ordinary or law-abiding citizenry. War tribunal consequences of a verified industrial accident could not possibly have weighed on their act of firmly concealing such a truth by killing Mochtar. Had the Klender event actually been an accident, Mochtar would very likely have received the requested clemency and survived the war. But he did not. Why? It is implausible that the Japanese killed Mochtar with no motive but spite—he hadn't done anything to earn it beyond his successful technical assault on Hideyo Noguchi's work two decades earlier.

The technical facts of tetanus and its vaccination, taken with the actions of the Japanese as the war drew to a bitter close, permit us to confidently reject accident as the cause of death of the romusha at Klender. This leaves us with only one likely explanation: deliberate contamination of the vaccine with tetanus toxin by the Japanese medical men at Bandung. Had they done so, Yamamoto would know of it and act firmly to protect those responsible for it (including himself). Such an accounting aligns with known Japanese state of mind and official actions at that late hour of the Pacific War.

This explanation, however, requires discovering Japanese motivation for doing so. Why would they put deadly toxin into vaccine ampoules and kill hundreds of Indonesians working on their behalf?

Exploration of this key question leads us to examine courtroom transcripts of the war tribunal proceedings against three Japanese navy men charged with murdering fifteen condemned Indonesian prisoners with tetanus toxin in Surabaya in February and March 1945.

The event at Surabaya shares important characteristics with the murders at Klender, although they are not directly linked. The navy men being tried in 1951 expressed nothing indicating awareness of what had happened at Klender in 1944, six months before carrying out their own experiment, nor did any officer of the tribunal. We know the navy men communicated with and even visited the Japanese army men at Bandung in a desperate (and futile) attempt to obtain stocks of tetanus antiplasma. The army men apparently made no mention of tetanus toxoid or the event at Klender. A fuller consideration of this interaction and its relevance to understanding both events may come with first examining the nuances of army-navy subcultures within the Imperial Japanese armed forces and their strategic posture in early 1945.

Army–Navy Games: Java 1945

When the Japanese occupied the East Indies, they created three administrative military zones. The Twenty-fifth Army managed Sumatra, the Sixteenth Army handled almost all of Java (including Surabaya), and the navy managed all else in the former colony. In most modern militaries, armies and navies represent competing and often mutually hostile subcultures. This was certainly true in the empire of Japan. As a general rule, one service depended upon the other when necessity forced it. As many Indonesian elites note in their memoirs of the occupation, the Japanese navy men tended to be more gentlemanly, intellectual, and less rabidly nationalistic than their army counterparts. However, to many ordinary Indonesians and Allied prisoners of war who experienced either culture, such distinction was either not obvious or else irrelevant. The army had no monopoly on conspicuous brutality. Some of the most heinous mass murders in occupied Indonesia would be at the hands of the navy men managing Borneo and all other outer islands in the archipelago.

The Japanese navy, within the army areas of responsibility on Java, was largely confined to the important seaports of Surabaya and Jakarta. These navy enclaves attended to the business of their ships, supplies, and people with their own resources. Unlike Allied forces, having continuous streams of supplies from home providing every need, Japanese forces in conquered lands were largely left to fend for themselves, even at the pinnacle of Imperial might in July 1942.

The deployment orders explicitly expressed this aspect of their mission: find what you require, take it, and put it to work in completing your military mission. Distinct military units had to be resourceful and, very often, cruelly rapacious in maintaining their readiness. No other units in the same area, much less distant Tokyo, could be depended upon for vital resources.

Navy enclaves would not count on army ingenuity and generosity in meeting these needs. They would strive very hard for self-sufficiency, as ordered. Nonetheless, there would be things the navy would have to ask the army to deliver, like rice from the army-managed interior. Likewise, the army would sometimes require things the navy could deliver, like goods from home and sea transport. So they cooperated, reluctantly, on essential needs.

As Allied command of the seas strangled supply lines to Java almost completely by early 1945, the army would likely have become less sympathetic to providing their own precious and dwindling resources for supporting the diminishingly useful navy. As the probability of Allied landings in the East Indies grew to misplaced certainty, each service, and even individual units within them, began to brace for the bloody struggle they had been ordered to carry out. They collected and hoarded the materials they would need.

Thus was the setting for an event that occurred in Surabaya in 1945 that bears directly upon Japanese motivation in the Mochtar affair.

Nakamura War Crime Tribunal: Manus Island, Papua New Guinea, 1951

Navy Captain Nakamura Hirosato was an ear, nose, and throat physician serving as the chief surgeon of the Second South Seas Expeditionary Fleet based at Surabaya. He had arrived for duty in November 1944. From March 20 to April 2, 1951, Nakamura stood trial under Australian military tribunal authority at Manus Island, Papua New Guinea, for the murder of fifteen Indonesians at a Surabaya prison in early 1945.[6]

Along with his two codefendants, Vice Adm. Shibata Yaichiro, Commander of the Fleet and Nakamura's direct superior, and Maj.

Tatsuzaki Ei, fleet legal officer, Nakamura was charged on three counts: the war crime of murder, the war crime of unlawful killing, and the mistreatment of native inhabitants of occupied territories.

Shibata was acquitted on all counts. Tatsuzaki, who made the condemned prisoners available for medical experimentation, was convicted on the second count of unlawful killing and sentenced to three years imprisonment, later commuted to just one year. Nakamura was also convicted of the second count and acquitted of the first and third counts. He would serve the full four-year imprisonment.

The basis for the apparent leniency shown these men may be gleaned by a careful reading of the trial transcripts. The deaths they caused indeed resulted from an immoral and illegal medical experiment, but their guilt was mitigated by the care exercised in ensuring the experiment would be minimally dangerous and the vigorous clinical efforts taken to save lives once it became clear that the experiment had failed. Nakamura had not intended to kill the prisoners and expressed his deep surprise and remorse at the outcome of his experiment. Technical incompetence caused the deaths, and in a strictly legal sense the criminality came with such negligence and in failing to obtain the informed consent of the prisoners.

The medical crime at Surabaya involved an experimental tetanus toxoid vaccination of seventeen natives of Lombok who were imprisoned at Surabaya and sentenced to death for their involvement in the murder of a Japanese officer and several Lombok residents. The Australian tribunal court deemed those convictions verified by fact and the sentences meted out as legal.

Although Nakamura, as chief surgeon of the fleet, took the legal brunt of responsibility for this experiment, other officers actually carried out the experiment: Surgeon Lt. Cmdr. Ide Manasori, chief of the Clinical Research Division, and Dr. Sugiura Yasumasa, a tetanus expert flown in from Tokyo for this project. These men were named as the parties who did the experimental work on the tetanus vaccine. They were not charged with any crime.

At a laboratory facility several kilometers from the naval hospital at Surabaya, Ide and Sugiura worked feverishly to prepare tetanus toxoid for vaccination. They ran thorough experiments in guinea pigs, measuring the lethal dose of toxin in control and vaccinated animals, essentially as described by the standard protocols already detailed. They determined that two vaccinations with toxoid increased the minimal lethal dose (MLD) of toxin 500-fold. Thus they felt they had created a product for vaccination that would provide very good protective efficacy against naturally acquired tetanus.

These military scientists were focused on vaccinating Japanese troops before the anticipated Allied landings and the heavy bloodshed that would follow. The landings were considered to be possible at any moment and virtually certain within a few months. They had run out of time to properly test their vaccine in cohorts of consenting vaccinated and unvaccinated people and then recording the rates of occurrence of naturally acquired tetanus in both groups. This would have been, by the ethical standards of the day, the proper way of testing the efficacy of an experimental vaccine against tetanus in human subjects. It also would have required many tens of thousands of volunteers and at least several years. This was beyond the capacity and timeframe of the Japanese navy scientists at Surabaya.

At a Second Expeditionary Navy staff meeting chaired by Shibata, Nakamura learned of seventeen Indonesians being held in the prison in Surabaya awaiting execution. After some internal discussion and several weeks of debate, Nakamura's scientists were given access to the condemned men.

All of the Japanese men involved described, at least in hindsight of their accountability, considering the clinical safety of the condemned men. The legal officer, Tatsuzaki, took a great deal of persuading. He pointed out the lack of a legal basis for doing the experiment and suffered legal anxiety over its conduct.

His testimony reads, "Then I told him [Nakamura] that as a lawyer I was of the opinion that I could not agree with him [on using the prisoners in an experiment] because testing of medicine is not provided for in the law, but owing to the circumstances, I told him I would consider it."

The defense counsel asked, "Did you give your consent or not?"

"No, I did not give it."

"And then what happened?"

Tatsuzaki replied, "The reason for not giving my consent to the Adjutant [to make the prisoners available for experimentation] was that, although I knew that their opinion as doctors was not wrong, to make a test on prisoners is not provided in the law, and therefore I was at a loss in making a decision."

Later he continued, "As a lawyer I could not consent to what was not prescribed, and it was over this inconsistency that I was worried for a few days."

Only the assurance of safety from the medical men and the military strategic need to conduct the experiment brought Tatsuzaki around to agreement. With professional reluctance, he surrendered access to the condemned men.

The court later asked Tatsuzaki if the prisoners had been offered the opportunity to volunteer for the experiment. He replied, "It was not because I did not think about the matter, but as the natives were less intelligent I thought they would not understand the matter, and steps were not taken to explain it to them."

The court retorted, "Well at any rate, did this enter your mind; that if the nature of the experiment were truthfully explained to the natives and their consent obtained after that explanation, no one could have anything to say about your conduct in this matter?" By today's standards of ethical conduct in research, even the informed consent of the prisoners would be dubious and unacceptable. People in no position to decline cannot be offered the opportunity to volunteer, and facing death by execution is very clearly such a position.

Shibata was also queried on the issue of informed consent, and his answers shed light on the thinking of the Japanese military men on this point.

The prosecutor asked Shibata, "Did you see anything wrong in the use of these condemned prisoners as subjects for experiment?"

"Yes, I thought it was wrong for them to use the condemned prisoners without first obtaining my permission."

"Without first obtaining your permission?"

"Officers attached to Headquarters should not use such condemned prisoners on their own discretion."

"But do you not consider it wrong that condemned prisoners should be used without their permission?"

One can almost see the admiral pausing in thought and finally realizing the point. He answered, "I thought it was wrong."

Modus Operandi

The Experiment: Surabaya, late January 1945 to early March 1945

The experiment was simple in concept. Vaccinate the prisoners with tetanus toxoid and then later inject them with purified toxin. Survival with that toxin challenge would prove the vaccine effective. All seventeen condemned prisoners received two vaccinations, a prime and a boost, in vaccine terminology, at a two-week interval. None suffered any serious effects and after an additional two weeks all were noted to be in good health. At this point they were divided into three toxin challenge groups: two times, one time, and one half times the estimated lethal dose of toxin. They had worked these doses out in unvaccinated horses (not guinea pig MLDS).

At trial, Nakamura pointed to the protection in guinea pigs reaching 500 times the lethal dose. They considered the two times lethal dose (for a horse) administered to the prisoners as being well within the margin of safety for even a slightly effective vaccine. He described careful thought in arriving at the challenge doses of toxin, striving to strike a balance between a credible test of vaccine efficacy against the safety of the subjects.

Beginning at about four days after injection with toxin, the first prisoner began to exhibit loss of appetite and an agitated state of mind. Ide examined his subjects and ordered their transfer from the prison to a hospital for observation. Three days later all of them had fallen ill, and after four more days of intensive care that included infusions of precious antitoxin serum, fifteen were dead. The two survivors allowed to fully recover in hospital were then returned to the prison and promptly executed.

The testimony given by the Japanese scientists appears to reflect genuine surprise and disappointment by the outcome of their experiment. They had worked within what they considered good safety margins. They had administered the same dosing regimen applied to the animals: vaccination; wait two weeks; booster shot; wait two more weeks; challenge with toxin. In retrospect, they realized that their extrapolation of data from animals to humans—as though a perfect correlation existed—was wishful thinking, driven by their desire to deploy their vaccine as quickly as possible. No one can know exactly what went wrong, but a combination of inadequate vaccination by dose or preparation of toxoid, along with too brief an interval between booster and challenge with toxin, may explain the fate of their victims.

Nakamura and Ide also expressed doubts about their calculations of minimum lethal dose or in their determination of toxin concentration in their challenge preparations. That is, the challenge perhaps contained far more toxin than they had reckoned. There was no mention of the weight of the horses used to derive their lethal dose numbers, or if they had extrapolated to the weight of the prisoners. The data constituted the basis of these doubts: among the prisoners challenged with 0.5MLD, none survived, whereas one of the two survivors had allegedly received the 2.0MLD challenge.

The reaction of the navy men to the onset of illness and eventually death among their test subjects demonstrates the seriousness they attached to the matter. Nakamura and Tatsuzaki immediately reported in person to Shibata, as it became clear the prisoners were ill and at risk of death. Consternation and worry was focused on the law rather than on the apparent inadequacy of their manufactured vaccine against tetanus. Shibata ordered them to do everything possible to save the stricken prisoners.

The design and outcome of this morally grotesque and technically shabby experiment is not the most relevant issue with respect to the Mochtar affair. Important insights into the event at Klender arise, instead, from examining what drove these Japanese navy men to invest their precious resources and legal risk in the frantic endeavor to produce a tetanus vaccine.

Military Medicine

Nakamura explained to the tribunal that he aimed to vaccinate more than 100,000 Japanese troops in preparation for the anticipated battle for the archipelago. His medical responsibility was to the Japanese navy troops scattered across the archipelago rather than to the Sixteenth Army troops on Java under the responsibility of the Japanese Army men at Jakarta and Bandung. Tetanus represented a serious threat to battlefield injured, and successful vaccination against it would dramatically improve survival rates. We know Nakamura acted decisively to meet that responsibility, and we believe his army counterparts did the same for their troops on Java.

Modus Operandi

As has been explained, the tetanus bacillus requires an environment free of oxygen in order to emerge from its hard capsule and begin producing toxin. The evolutionary advantage of this toxin is unclear. Its deadly effects may be either an unhappy coincidence or a strategy for producing a largely oxygen-free corpse suited to growth.

The microenvironments of deep wounds, with chunks of tissue cut off from oxygen supply, provide pockets where the bacterium can thrive. Battlefield injuries and abundant soil contamination represent a veritable nursery for *C. tetani*. Before the advent of toxoid vaccine, military doctors were long familiar with the specific signs and the agonizing deaths of tetanus victims. The 1809 painting of the British soldier dying of tetanus after surviving gunshot wounds was rendered by Sir Charles Bell, an army surgeon.

How serious of a military medicine problem would the lack of tetanus antitoxin or toxoid vaccine be? Tetanus attack rates from wars before the advent of either antitetanus plasma or tetanus toxoid provide a quick snapshot of the weight of the problem and of the relief provided by these technologies. In the 1860s, during the American Civil War, before tetanus antitoxin was available, 205 tetanus fatalities occurred per 100,000 wounded soldiers. The availability of antitoxin plasma during World War I reduced this rate to 16 tetanus deaths per 100,000 wounded soldiers. During World War II, American military forces were almost all vaccinated with toxoid vaccine, and they experienced only 0.44 cases per 100,000 wounded.[7] The protective efficacy of antitoxin plasma administered to wounded soldiers may thus be estimated at 92 percent and of toxoid vaccination at 99.8 percent. The strategic imperative, at least in the mind of a military physician, would indeed be great.

Tetanus toxoid was twenty-year-old technology at the outbreak of World War II, and by 1942 Allied forces were routinely vaccinated with tetanus toxoid. This was not so among Japanese troops. Their military medical research infrastructure lagged behind that of the Allies. Japanese military medical doctrine prescribed only the use of antitoxin serum administered to the wounded.

Nakamura testified that he first tried to meet anticipated combat needs for tetanus antitoxin plasma, but without success. Importation from Japan was out of the question. Few ships were surviving the journey by early 1945. He testified to contacting the Japanese army laboratory at Bandung (the former Pasteur Institute) in January 1945 and again in May, requesting tetanus antitoxin plasma. He described receiving stocks sufficient for routine noncombat needs, but far less than required for the anticipated battle for the East Indies. The army had very little to spare, although Nakamura testified that the army offered abundant supplies of vaccines against cholera, typhus, dysentery, plague, and smallpox. He made no mention of an army tetanus toxoid vaccine.

In the context of the Mochtar affair, this simple fact is damning. A senior Japanese medical officer responsible for the health of more than 100,000 combat-ready troops facing imminent battle could not obtain tetanus prevention products from the army vaccine facility at Bandung. What explains the failure of Captain Nakamura to obtain tetanus toxoid vaccine from the army at Bandung? And if the army had it, why hoard the antitoxin plasma? It would appear they did not have the toxoid vaccine to offer.

This is Nakamura's testimony: "In December 1944 I contacted the osamu unit of the Japanese army for a supply of serums, and further, in January 1945 I contacted the army laboratory at Bandoeng, also for the purpose of obtaining serums from them, and further in May 1945 I again contacted both of these organs for a supply of serums."

The prosecutor asked: "What was the result of your exertions?"

Nakamura replied, "We were unable to get approval from the army."

This testimony is credible in that it would have little bearing upon the tribunal's judgment of Nakamura. The military urgency of the matter is clear in his efforts to obtain products from the army, and then striving to solve the problem by producing a toxoid vaccine. Further, the Japanese concerns regarding tetanus were perfectly rational in a military preventive medicine sense. Nakamura's testimony reveals the medical strategic position of the army men at Bandung with respect to the very same problem: they had limited supplies of antitoxin plasma and no toxoid vaccine product.

This is damning because the army men at Bandung possessed and successfully operated one of the most technically and industrially advanced vaccine production facilities in Southeast Asia. What

Modus Operandi

had they been doing to deal with the urgent tetanus prevention problem? It is highly improbable that those ideally placed and equipped army scientists did nothing whatsoever.

If they had been as active as Nakamura, who had vastly less expertise and production capacities, and followed his rational and technically appropriate (but amoral) approach to the problem, a toxoid vaccine would have been in development at Bandung. The catastrophe at Klender would explain their empty-handedness when Nakamura came calling for solutions to his tetanus problem in January 1945. The toxoid vaccine product used at Klender, if they still possessed it, would certainly not be considered useable. The dire political and legal consequences of their technical failure likely prohibited correcting it and conducting further testing of the product on human guinea pigs. The few bags of antitoxin plasma provided to Nakamura were almost certainly all they could offer.

Something had caused the Japanese army men at Bandung to fail in meeting a critical military medical requirement for combat readiness and the survival of their wounded soldiers. That something could not have been inadequate know-how, poor facilities, or a lack of commitment to the task. We cannot know with certainty what that was, but the disastrous outcome to a medical experiment at Klender is a rational and wholly plausible explanation.

The Case for Medical Experimentation at Klender

The hypothesis of industrial accident as the cause of death in the vaccinated romusha at Klender has already been firmly rejected, but this conclusion bears some consideration in light of Nakamura's testimony. He revealed the army at Bandung having limited tetanus antitoxin plasma and thus motivation for pursuing a tetanus toxoid solution to that problem. Further, Nakamura had been offered limitless supplies of other vaccines, including TCD (typhoid, cholera, dysentery). Recall that Jatman described a failed batch of TCD plus tetanus toxoid being set aside for disposal immediately before the occupation. This led to speculation about that batch being put into the romusha at Klender in 1944. Nakamura's testimony tends to paint such a scenario as improbable: there were abundant supplies of TCD vaccine at Bandung and therefore no need to rummage for it.

We know that immediately before the Japanese invasion of Java the KNIL had ordered the Dutch scientists at Pasteur Institute to develop a toxoid vaccine for formulation with the standard TCD product. The Dutch did so despite the long-standing ability to produce antitoxin plasma. The military medical men within KNIL obviously deemed that therapy inadequate and ordered the toxoid product. The Dutch scientists at Bandung apparently had already started down that path when the Japanese arrived. That data would end up in the hands of the Japanese military medical men at Boeki Kenkyujo.

The key question is whether the Japanese indeed embarked on the same endeavor. If they did not, the hypothesis of experiment at Klender must be dismissed. If they did, the experiment almost certainly took place. The hypothetical linkage of the event at Klender with an experiment aimed at proving the efficacy of a tetanus toxoid vaccine must be examined against what is known with certainty. In other words, does an experiment at Klender rationally align with the known facts?

An analysis of such alignment may be constructed by listing the suppositions required in accepting that the Japanese indeed experimented at Klender. Under each, let us consider the consistency of the known facts with the supposition:

The Japanese at Bandung would have been driven to develop a tetanus toxoid vaccine.

The military situation demanded this. Ordered to defend their hold on Java by force of mortal combat, and anticipating Allied invasion, they would have been ordered to develop and produce toxoid vaccines, as the KNIL had ordered their Dutch predecessors to do. The actions and testimony of the Japanese navy men at Surabaya affirms that strategic imperative. It is also known that the army men at Bandung had limited supplies of the inferior option of antitoxin plasma.

The Japanese at Bandung had the capacity to develop a tetanus toxoid vaccine.

There is no question regarding this supposition. The Pasteur Institute run by the Japanese army was the most technically advanced and equipped vaccine development and manufacturing facility in Southeast Asia. The Pasteur Institute had not only been in the early stages of tetanus toxoid vaccine development, but it also had a decades-old tetanus toxin production capacity (for its industrial production of antitoxin plasma). Everything required was on hand, likely including the Dutch records of their progress on their incomplete tetanus toxoid project.

The Japanese at Bandung would overcome the abhorrent ethics of testing the efficacy of their product by putting toxin into the romusha.

The private view of the Japanese on the romusha as disposable commodities, demonstrated when out of sight of the Indonesian masses, is perfectly consistent with their use of the romusha as human guinea pigs (and careful concealment of such). Even setting aside the broader immoral and sadistic medical experiments of Unit 731 in China and elsewhere, the example of the navy men at Surabaya certainly demonstrates a willingness to risk the lives of medical subjects in the interest of the military medical strategic imperative. Like those navy men, the Japanese army scientists at Bandung would desire evidence of protective efficacy before ramping up a production run of several hundred thousand doses. Unlike their Dutch predecessors, the Japanese at Bandung did not routinely undertake experimental development of vaccines. Their menu of vaccines for public consumption included nothing beyond that already under proven industrial production when they arrived. Their confidence in their own experimental vaccine would not be solid with tetanus toxoid.

The Japanese at Bandung would want to test their vaccine at Klender.

It is difficult to imagine a better population in which to do so. The romusha at Klender were available by the hundreds, in easy reach, confined to that location, pliant to orders, relatively healthy, and receiving legitimate vaccinations made by the facility at Bandung on a routine basis. They could conduct the experiment without arousing suspicion.

The Japanese at Bandung had access to the romusha at Klender.

No record or testimony places the Japanese army medical men from Bandung at Klender. The Japanese army men managing the camp would not have been in the direct chain of command of those at the vaccine facility at Bandung. They could not simply show up and demand romusha for injections, even if they outranked the keepers at the camp. That access would likely only come with the consent of high command at Jakarta. No evidence exists of such consent, but, as in Surabaya, access could be obtained through successfully explaining the strategic necessity and the improbability of harm in granting it.

The Japanese army provided and had control over the vaccines administered to the doomed romusha at Klender.

This would have to be true for the conduct of an experiment involving three injections separated by at least two weeks—prime and then boost with the experimental toxoid vaccine, followed by challenge with unadulterated purified tetanus toxin. While testimony shows that the municipal health service (headed by Dr. Marzoeki) used its own stocks of vaccines from Bandung when ordered to routinely vaccinate romusha at Klender, we know in the instance of the fatal vaccine that this routine was broken. When Dr. Marzoeki was tasked with administering the injections by the Japanese authorities, he recorded that he was instructed by the Japanese army to bring no supplies to Klender. They explained to him that the vaccines would be supplied on site. This was not routine. Marzoeki's wife, Corrie, affirmed this important point in her memoir of the event: "One morning Mars [Marzoeki] got a phone call from the military office to send some physicians and nurses to assist in the immunization program [at Klender], but without any serum because that would be available on location." The Japanese controlled the ampoules used to inject the romusha that died a week later. Moreover it may be seen that the Japanese army exercised control over the general vaccination of romusha—the municipal health service vaccinated romusha only when ordered to do so by the Japanese.

The Japanese at Bandung considered the experiment at Klender low risk.

Several lines of evidence support this supposition. They would not have deliberately killed the romusha, as the fact of their deaths and its fallout demonstrated. Tetanus toxin had to be placed in those vaccinations with the earnest belief that it would cause no harm. As with the navy men at Surabaya, it is almost certain that the deaths due to tetanus intoxication came as a shocking, frightening, and bitter technical failure. The Japanese clearly were not prepared for the calamity. In the first day, events unfolded out of the control of the Japanese. They needed precious hours to respond and then quickly acted to sanitize the disaster.

The Japanese at Jakarta acted to conceal the truth of what happened at Klender.

This is beyond any reasoned doubt. The obviously conjured act of sabotage speaks for itself on this supposition. Why they did so, and to such physically brutal and politically risky extremes, bears directly on the hypothesis of medical experiment. In the absence of even a remote possibility of an embarrassing industrial accident, we are left with the conclusion that their actions were aimed at concealing some grievous wrongdoing on their part. The most likely explanation is the testing of the efficacy of their experimental tetanus toxoid vaccine with the same misplaced confidence shown at Surabaya, and inadvertently killing nine hundred young Indonesian men.

We consider the suppositions needed to impose a medical experiment as the basis of the event at Klender as fully compatible with the known facts of the catastrophe. There is no fact known to us that even remotely begins to nullify that possibility. Had we discovered possibly exculpatory evidence, it would have been described.

In the English summary of his memoir of the Mochtar affair, Ali Hanafiah concludes:

What had really happened was as follows:

Chotypa [TCD] vaccines, including the ones applied in Klender, were produced by the Pasteur Institute in Bandung, which at the time had been taken over by the Japanese Health Authorities. Before the war, the institute had failed to process anatoxin [toxoid vaccine].

The Japanese themselves performed an experiment with tetanus anatoxin which proved fatal.

The group accused never existed.[8]

Almost forty years ago, and thirty years after the event, Hanafiah arrived at conclusions effectively mirroring our own. His own first-hand experience, decades of deliberation, and interviews of other victims led to the same explanation of experiment for the deaths of the romusha victims. The supposition base of Hanafiah's argument or perhaps its unexplained technical nuance presumably accounts for the persistence of the hypothesis of industrial accident to explain the Klender calamity in Indonesia and abroad to the present day.

The Experiment at Klender

The testing of an experimental tetanus toxoid vaccine in the romusha at Klender by the Japanese army men at Bandung is a hypothesis. The evidence supporting it is circumstantial, albeit substantial and compelling, in our opinion. A final argument for its veracity in representing the likely truth and consistency with known facts may best be presented as a hypothetical reconstruction of the event.

In early 1944 the looming possibility of an Allied invasion of Java launched from Australia or New Guinea elicited strategy, tactics, and actions from the Japanese military occupation government. Surface shipping of men and materiel from elsewhere in the empire—especially from distant Japan—became increasingly hazardous, infrequent, and improbable. Allied war strategy had aimed for precisely this in their single-minded beeline for Tokyo and those holding the reins of Imperial power. The Sixteenth Army and Navy partners looked inward for their military requirements. One small but significant facet of those needs was a military medical solution for the threat of tetanus to wounded soldiers. They anticipated coping with many thousands wounded.

Scientists in Japan may have been producing tetanus toxoid vaccine for military use by 1944, but they had limited options in getting it to the southern fringe of their empire. The navy flying in a tetanus expert from Japan to Surabaya (Dr. Sugiura) attests to the availability of such expertise and the importance attached to accessing it by the most practical means. The army command in Jakarta likely ordered their subordinates at Boeki Kenkyujo in Bandung to develop and ramp up production of tetanus vaccine.

The army scientists at Bandung faced the challenge of a technical task they had not yet undertaken—developing a new vaccine rather than simply turning the production cogs for vaccines developed and perfected by the Dutch masters of this precise technology. They naturally looked to the records of the uncompleted project launched by the Dutch in the months preceding their invasion. The Dutch had been ordered to augment the TCD vaccine with tetanus toxoid. The Japanese would have picked up that work where the Dutch left off, likely sparing them months of effort and increasing their chances of success.

Like their navy counterparts in Surabaya, the Japanese at Bandung would probably quickly and effectively optimize tetanus toxoid production into a safe, immunogenic, and effective (in animals) vaccine product. They would have known this, as did the navy men, by standard tests in guinea pigs. They would also have been rationally skeptical of translating such formulations directly to humans. A production run and administration of several hundred thousand potentially faulty vaccinations would require a great deal of time and precious resources, not to mention the lives of wounded Japanese soldiers lost to tetanus. It is doubtful they would have found tests in macaques fully reassuring against such a catastrophic failure.

They would explore technical solutions to this uncertainty and settle upon an experiment to demonstrate with virtual certainty that vaccinated Japanese troops, once wounded in combat, would not be lost to tetanus. They would have then known, with equal certitude, that this requires vaccinating humans with their experimental toxoid formulation and then challenging them with natural, purified tetanus toxin. They needed, almost literally in this technical context, human guinea pigs. The Japanese army medical men at Bandung, some of them perhaps veterans of the ghastly Unit 731 experiments in China, would not blink at such a comparatively benign experiment. The human guinea pigs needed were fully expected to survive such experimentation.

Their scientific sights were set on the romusha at Klender. They could immunize these men with vaccines labeled the standard TCD formulation. The addition of toxoid, per Dutch data on that formulation, for the immunizations followed by a third vaccination with TCD containing pure tetanus toxin (for which no Dutch data would be available) would do. The experiment could be done under complete cover of routine vaccination, and done so with complete control and supervision of the subjects. They would have written up a secret protocol for this decisive and critical experiment.

The commander at Boeki Kenkyujo, as Nakamura had done in Surabaya, would have taken the plan to his commander in Jakarta for approval, if for no other reason than to obtain access to the romusha at Klender. The protocol probably didn't reach the level of Yamamoto (head of the military occupation), as he would have likely delegated that responsibility to an officer of general rank. Permission to proceed, as in Surabaya, would have been a carefully weighed decision made only with the most confident reassurances from the experts at Bandung. Because the experiment appears to have been executed, we may presume such permission was obtained.

The crucial technical decision in that experiment was the dose of toxin with which to challenge the immunized romusha. As we can see with the experiment in Surabaya, this was a vexing problem. The scientists had no precedent data upon which to draw. They were in a technical sense on unexplored ground. They had to work this out for themselves. The community of medical science, even in the early twentieth century, did not consider putting pure toxin at any dose into immunized human subjects remotely moral or ethically acceptable. The Japanese army men at Bandung, rising above such obstacles, were on their own to develop the technical solution to this arrangement.

Beyond understanding that their technical solution was fatally flawed, we cannot know what it was or how they derived it. We can only rationally suppose that they earnestly believed it had been worked out satisfactorily. They prepared TCD vaccines with the dose of tetanus toxin deemed sufficient to evaluate the efficacy of their toxoid vaccine. Those ampoules awaited the Indonesian doctors administering what they thought were routine TCD vaccinations to the romusha at Klender.

The scale of their simple experiment, hundreds of men, hints strongly at the misplaced confidence of the men conducting it. Far more modest numbers would have sufficed. That confidence and their apparent desire to conceal that it had been done at all, likely explains the lack of control at the onset of the disastrous events at Klender. The Japanese military managers of the camp seem to have been completely unaware of what had actually taken place. They permitted Indonesian medical first responders into the camp and even handed over patients and empty ampoules to them. When those in the know finally understood what was happening, they sealed the camp and acted to secure documentary evidence created at the hospital in Jakarta.

The experiment failed, probably for the same reasons it would fail again in Surabaya six months later. The subjects of this experiment, though almost certainly immunized with an adequate toxoid vaccine prior to challenge, had likely received doses of toxin far in excess of that capable of preventing acute tetanus in immunized people. The lingering presence of viable toxin in tissues extracted from the corpses of people injected about a week earlier (demonstrated by Jatman at the Eijkman) hints at a relatively massive dose. This "depot effect" of biological materials sitting in the flesh after injection is by no means long lasting under ordinary circumstances. What remained in those tissues was probably a small fraction of what had been injected the week before.

The Japanese response to this calamity has been explained in previous chapters. That response is factual and not hypothetical. They crudely painted Achmad Mochtar as a saboteur and mass murderer. How they actually caused the deaths of the romusha at Klender compelled them to conceal it with an elaborate lie. This, too, is factual rather than hypothetical.

Fear of the political consequences of the experiment at Klender, had its nature become known in August 1944, has been explained. Such fear likely motivated the Japanese early in their management of the disaster. Mochtar's confession and conviction spared the Japanese and their elite nationalist friends from potentially calamitous political fallout. The knowledge that the romusha had been subjected to a lethal medical experiment, and that nationalist leaders had endorsed and promoted their use by the Japanese, would have eroded their political base, perhaps to the point of collapse. Once that risk had been managed, and the war pressed on in the direction of their defeat, Japanese worries would shift to legal consequences.

Allied discovery of such an experiment at Klender probably would have meant sentences of death to those who carried it out. The Australian tribunal showed relative leniency to Nakamura. His remorse, his technical (although incompetent) safety measures, the heroic efforts to save the lives of the stricken research subjects, and the fact that the prisoners were condemned and natives rather than POWs were all cited as mitigating factors. Other war tribunals were not so forgiving. For example, the German malariologist Klaus Schilling experimented with malaria vaccines on Dachau inmates, and thirty to forty died of induced malaria: Schilling and many other Nazi doctors were tried, convicted and hung.[9] The murder of nine hundred men not otherwise condemned, and with almost no Japanese effort to save their lives, would offer little mitigation of guilt.

Though the Japanese in Jakarta of mid-1945 could not know of the verdicts of either Nakamura or Schilling, we know they saw war tribunals in their future. The American government had communicated to the government of Japan—in the form of diplomatic protest via the Swiss mission in Tokyo—some of its evidence of atrocities committed by the Japanese beginning as early as 1942. As has been explained, the Japanese high command in Tokyo ordered the destruction of incriminating evidence in the months leading up to surrender. The mien of the Japanese at the time of Mochtar's execution was evasion of accountability for war crimes.

The Japanese army medical men at Bandung would escape prosecution for the dead romusha at Klender with the aid of Mochtar's false confession. It secured not only the life and liberty of Mochtar's friends but also those of his false accusers. It is nearly certain that all beneficiaries who had worn the Japanese army uniform in Bandung during the occupation are now deceased after living their lives free of accountability for their crime. They accepted Mochtar's gift of life and liberty with no known acknowledgment of gratitude or admission of wrongdoing. They perhaps considered Mochtar and the romusha to have been victims of the Allies whose colonial imperialism required the Japanese to go to war to defend their homeland. In this very simple dichotomy of thoughts and actions—selfish versus selfless—we find the purest expression of the human spirit as wicked or virtuous.

Ancol, 3 July 1945

The only known account of Mochtar's execution comes from Mohammad Hatta, as described by Abu Hanifah:

> Hatta told me that a Japanese from Hawaii, a Nisei scientist, visited him at his home. This man was busy writing a book about the Pacific War. He was also interested in the atrocities committed during the war. So he went to Japan to study war documents and talk to war veterans. It seemed there existed a small book, a diary of a Japanese intelligence officer, in which there were notes about the execution of well-known people in the places where this man had served. He saw there the name of Professor Mochtar and he read the story of the execution. It seemed that Dr. Mochtar was first beheaded and then they drove a steam roller over his body and put the remains in a truck together with other bodies and buried them all in a mass grave somewhere in the swamps near the coast.[10]

That would be the mass grave at Ancol, just forty meters from the sea. We harbor doubts about the dramatic and horrifying steamroller mentioned here, but do not dismiss it entirely. The execution ground was an unlikely site for such equipment, and the Japanese would have had little or no known motivation for such a barbaric and public display at that very late stage of their occupation. Hanifah seems given to some degree of exaggeration in his emotional recollections and accounting of the martyrdom suffered by his dear uncle.

Today the tree under which the Japanese executed prisoners, very probably including Mochtar, stands at the edge of the Dutch-Indonesian cemetery, Ereveld Ancol. The tree is dead. Cement at its base prevents it from falling over. The branches are trimmed back and it has been thoroughly shellacked. A brass plate is embedded in its trunk with a poem entitled "Hemelboom" (Heaven Tree).

> They shall not grow old
> As we that are left grow old:
> Age shall not weary them,
> Nor the years condemn.
> At the going down of the sun
> And in the morning
> We shall remember them
> We shall remember them

Though not cited on the tree, this is an excerpt from Laurence Binyon's poem "For the Fallen," published in 1914.[11]

Achmad Mochtar laid down his life at that tree, surrendering it so that others would live. Simon Flexner, in his stirring tribute to Hideyo Noguchi in *Science* magazine in 1929, suggested that the spirit of science and Noguchi's love of his fellow man would surely reside at the enshrined place of his birth and wretched upbringing. It does, without qualification or caveat. We suggest the wretched tree at Ancol should similarly stand for the deep humanity of Achmad Mochtar and his countless fellow victims of the inhumanity embodied in the selfish and misguided aspirations of a poisoned group identity, be it national, racial, religious, or any other. This, too, is the spirit of science. Achmad Mochtar left us its lessons to absorb and understand. These two men, Noguchi and Mochtar, though they were temporal adversaries in science and national identity, stand together in the barest and most honest expressions of true humanity. We can and should learn from both of these exemplary men.

TWELVE

Legacy

To Kill an Institute

The Japanese apparently made no declaration or notification of Mochtar's execution. They just registered his name in their dreadful log at Ancol and moved on to other ugly business. His family eventually realized that he would never return. The same was true at his institute among the very few colleagues remaining. A painful uncertainty of his innocence in the slaughter at Klender lingered with the grief of his loss. Certainty of his innocence also would dawn very slowly and quietly.

The fortunes of the Eijkman Institute sharply declined after Mochtar's murder, leading to formal closure twenty years later. Complex factors explain its demise, and there is risk of oversimplifying the matter. The two decades following 1945 were fraught with war, political conflict, social upheaval, and nationalist resentment toward relics of Dutch colonialism. Little was accomplished as legitimate scientific research, and the institute had declined to the role of a reference laboratory when it finally closed in 1965. We examine that decline in order to better grasp the cost of Mochtar's murder and of the Dutch attempt to reassert colonial domain over Indonesia after the Pacific War.

Within forty-eight hours of the Japanese surrender, Indonesia declared her independence a few blocks from the Eijkman Institute. Warfare in defense of that independence against the Dutch began in earnest a few months later. This new war made breathing life back into the Eijkman Institute both a low priority and an extremely improbable achievement. Bloody and vicious, that war poisoned for decades what had been collegial and productive relationships between Dutch and Indonesian scientists.

British troops were the first Allies to reach Indonesia. They were sent to disarm and repatriate the Japanese as well as to rescue prisoners and internees. But they found themselves unwittingly drawn into a rebellion as agents of the Dutch colonialists. Rebels had effectively seized control of Surabaya (Indonesia's second city) in eastern Java by October, and the British forces had to negotiate access to it. Negotiations took place and limited access was granted, but violence broke out, and a senior British officer (Brig. Gen. A.W.S. Mallaby) was killed. Impatient and angered by the general's death, the British launched a full-scale invasion of Surabaya in November 1945 under air and naval bombardment of the city. The poorly organized and barely equipped nationalists held half the city for an astonishing three weeks against this overpowering British force. The Battle of Surabaya cost six thousand rebel and civilian lives. The tenacity, ferocity, and courage of the rag-tag fighters at Surabaya helped persuade Britain to disengage from the conflict and assume neutrality in the war. Later Britain would stand in support of the rebel cause at the United Nations, where the battles of real consequence in this new war occurred.

Determined to remain masters of the archipelago, the Dutch pressed the nationalists militarily and ruthlessly, but the guerrilla tactics of their enemy rendered their superior arms and armor impotent. The nationalists typically attacked isolated military columns or outposts at sites of their choosing and advantage, inflicting damage and then vanishing into the civilian populace. Frustrated Dutch soldiers sank to vengeful massacres in villages suspected of supporting the nationalists.

Capt. Raymond Westerling commanded a counterinsurgency unit that went on a bloody rampage through villages near Makassar in the Celebes beginning in December 1946. In the ensuing two months, with escalating brutality, Westerling oversaw the murders of thousands of unarmed men, women, and children by rifle and bayonet. Estimates of the number murdered ranged from Westerling's 600 to the nationalists' 40,000.

Westerling returned to Batavia in March 1947 to a hero's welcome by the colonialists. His unit then slaughtered 430 boys and young men at Rawagede, West Java, on December 9, 1947. Under United Nations pressure to arrest Westerling as a war criminal, the Dutch permitted his escape. Westerling took refuge in Friesland, the Netherlands, where he took up the performing arts, including singing performances in Amsterdam. He passed away in 1987. The Dutch government steadfastly defended these massacres as legitimate "police actions" until September 2013, when it finally apologized to Indonesia for Westerling's massacres and offered compensation to survivors of the victims.

These wretched currents tugged hard at the underpinnings of the Eijkman Institute, which had been a successful and essentially collaborative Dutch-Indonesian scientific enterprise. The Dutch government dispatched new scientific staff in 1946. They were received with confusion and hostility from the strongly nationalist Indonesian medical community. There could be no collaborative work with the Dutch so long as they remained a foreign combatant enemy in the new republic.

In any event the institute had lost all of its leading scientists. The surviving interred Dutch, often deeply traumatized, mostly accepted repatriation to Holland (though some would later return to Batavia and the institute). The best Indonesian scientists, Mochtar and Raden Soesilo, had both been put to the sword. Among those tortured by the Kenpeitai, none are known to have returned to the institute with the exception of Ko Kiap Nio and Djoehana Wiradikarta. He had been vice director under Mochtar and succeeded him as director after the Japanese surrender. When the Dutch returned in 1946, they promptly replaced Djoehana with a Dutch scientist. Two other Dutch directors would follow until their final exit in 1950. Those crucial first years of potential recovery from the trauma of the Klender event were lost to deep animosities and renewed war.

The Japanese had gravely wounded the Eijkman Institute by their laundering of the Klender deaths, but it was the war conducted by the Dutch against Indonesia that sealed its fate.

The Indonesian national experience through the Pacific War and its immediate aftermath may be compared to the wartime experience of one Indonesian, Pak Ayal. In 1988 a coauthor of this book (JKB), a young lieutenant in the U.S. Navy, conducted malaria studies in northeastern Indonesian New Guinea. The driver of a vehicle he had leased, Bahar, explained that his *bapak*, Pak Ayal, wished to receive Lieutenant Baird at his home in Jayapura.[1] Pak Ayal had once been a navy man and was curious to meet another. Ayal, about seventy-five years of age, was warm and welcoming. The two sat on a veranda over cool drinks and enjoyed a breathtaking late afternoon view of the deep blue and vast Yos Sudarso Bay from Ayal's hilltop home in the "Dock 5" neighborhood of Jayapura. After casual conversation and getting to know one another, Ayal at length spoke of his naval experiences in nearly perfect English. This sailor had been around.

In early 1942 he was enlisted in the Dutch navy, serving as a steward on the light cruiser *de Ruyter* out of Surabaya. It was the command flagship of the doomed Allied flotilla in the Battle of the Java Sea. His gleaming modern ship having been "shot out from beneath me," Ayal clung to debris in the sea for many hours until he was rescued by a Japanese warship. Days later, he found himself in a POW camp near Surabaya. After he had been there for more than a year, the Japanese conscripted him for service in their navy. He served as steward on the Japanese heavy cruiser *Maya*. In October 1944, in the Battle of Leyte Gulf, Ayal's ship again disappeared from beneath him, and he floated in that sea until being rescued by a Japanese warship. The next day that ship too slipped beneath the waves. He was finally pulled from the sea by an American warship. A few weeks later he found himself again languishing in a POW camp, this one in northern Australia. At war's end he was repatriated to Indonesia and promptly recruited by the rebelling nationalists to operate a gunboat on the north coast of Java. After only a few weeks, the Dutch navy attacked and sank his gunboat. Ayal floated again in the Java Sea. He languished in a Dutch POW camp on Java until the end of the war in late 1949.

Ayal told his story with no apparent sense of the irony of it, as if the identities of those sinking his ships, pulling him from the sea, and holding him prisoner were of no consequence. He stood (or floated) both against and with each side of the warring combatants, like a bystander assimilated into the side that happened to surround him. He had no control over who owned his ships or who sank them. Asked about loyalties in the example of his gig with the nationalists, he explained accepting the assignment in the pragmatic terms of the aesthetics of the boat they offered—she was a beauty, and he wanted her. After his release from the Dutch POW camp, he saw another beauty and wanted her, too. He immigrated to Holland with his new Dutch wife. She later sank his matrimonial boat, and he washed up in Jayapura in the mid-1960s.

Indonesians had adapted and assimilated into the Dutch East Indies and did so with the Japanese occupiers. Like Ayal, the nation played the cards dealt them by global geopolitical dealers, displaying and capitalizing superb survival instincts and wits. They endured the foreign players on their national stage, and those players ultimately evicted each other from that stage. To the craven return of one, they barred the door using both bloody sacrifice and shrewd diplomacy.

Their victory over the brawny Dutch military mirrored the victorious little water buffalo of the Minangkabau—the Indonesian calf, craving the liberty denied it, poked and prodded the Dutch bull. Poorly armed but scrappy and savvy, the nationalists suffered defeat in a purely military sense but outwitted the Dutch on the postwar political stage. The most powerful victors of the Pacific War—the United States, Great Britain, and Australia—stood with the persuasive nationalists in resisting reassertion of colonial dominion in the East Indies. The Minangkabau Mohammad Hatta had represented the nationalist voice in that confrontation of intellects in the paddock of international diplomacy. The Dutch colonial bull fell over, mortally wounded.

Independence for all Asian nations from European colonialism was achieved by 1963 (Singapore), with remnant colonial enclaves lingering at East Timor and Macau (by the Portuguese until 1975 and 1999) and at Hong Kong (by the British until 1997). Some may argue that Guam at the southern extreme of the Marianas archipelago, existing as a U.S. territory since 1898 (setting aside the Japanese occupation of 1942–44), stands alone as a complex exception. Macau and Hong Kong became dominions of China, and East Timor had been annexed by Indonesian force of arms in the immediate wake of Portugal's precipitous exit. Indonesia relinquished control of East Timor in 1999, and it became an independent nation, Timor Leste, in 2002.

To Heal

After the Indonesians finally won their war for freedom in December 1949, the new minister of education, Dr. Abu Hanifah, warmly and wisely invited Dutch professors in the medical schools at Jakarta and Surabaya to remain in Indonesia. He wanted their help in training up the Indonesian professors who would assume their roles. In asking for such he was bluntly honest with them. At a meeting of the Faculty of Medicine, University of Indonesia at Salemba, he said:

> Gentlemen, I appeal to your love for your students and my beautiful country to help me out, at least for the first few years. However, I must tell you that I wouldn't like to see you involved in politics. Let me handle that end, and I'll give you complete freedom in the technical implementation of your work. If we have understood each other well, gentlemen, I would like to thank you for your work in the past and in advance for all our work in the future. I would like to convey to all of you my great thanks for your co-operation.[2]

Hanifah effectively invited the Dutch professors to join, in the sphere of medicine, in the task of building the Republic of Indonesia. He let them know this was a temporary arrangement, dispelling any delusional colonial thinking about permanency. The same invitation would perhaps have applied to Dutch scientists at the Eijkman Institute next door. Such bridge building was not to be, however. The government removed Hanifah. Domestic political enemies leveraged his warmth toward Dutch cooperation against him. Soekarno exported the nettlesome Hanifah as his ambassador to Brazil.

The new Republic still licked deep and painful wounds, and it had no appetite for Dutch in senior or influential positions, even temporary ones in medicine. Although many Dutch remained in Indonesia after independence, their roles in positions of technical leadership or influence were systematically eliminated.

Later, in 1958, the presence of even relatively low-level Dutch partners was almost entirely swept away in the wake of the political confrontation (and very nearly military, including the involvement of a
substantial naval force from the Soviet Union) on Netherlands New
Guinea. The Dutch had not ceded that territory in the 1949 treaty
acknowledging the Republic. They retained it as a colonial possession. Indonesian resentment at Dutch reluctance to exit this very
significant piece of "Indonesia Raya"–which amounts to more than
a quarter of Indonesia's land mass—ran extremely high.

The Dutch were again politically outmaneuvered in the United
Nations, this time on West New Guinea. They quit the colony in 1962.
Departing Dutch at Hollandia (now Jayapura) collected their dozens
of automobiles portside as they prepared to depart. The Dutch then
stacked the cars into a gigantic pile and set them ablaze. The cars
burned as they boarded their ships and sailed away.

This mutual animosity may in part explain the official closure of
the Eijkman Institute in 1965, prior to the communist coup d'état
attempt later that year. The Soekarno government, and perhaps the
public, would likely have viewed the institute as an unwanted relic
of Dutch colonialism.

Even worse, in his autobiography published in that tumultuous
year, Soekarno stubbornly insisted upon the guilt of Mochtar and
the entire staff of the Eijkman Institute in the murder of the romusha at Klender. Soekarno recalled a group of students challenging
him boldly on the loss of their beloved vice rector. "Why could you
not save Muchtar?" Soekarno answered, "Muchtar headed the laboratory which injected trainsful of romushas with anti-tetanus serum
prior to being shipped out. The vaccine was faulty. Within three
days tens of thousands died. The enormity of this was beyond what
I could offer the Japanese in return."[3]

That accounting is flawed in several conspicuous respects. Eijkman staff did not create or carry out the injections, and it was not, of
course, antitoxin plasma. Soekarno hedges the criminality with reference to faulty vaccine, perhaps reflecting what had already become
the most likely explanation among Mochtar's friends: the industrial accident hypothesis. Although no one knows the actual number of romusha killed at Klender, few would accept Soekarno's "tens

of thousands" of victims as remotely credible. He implicitly admits weighing the plea for clemency and rejecting its pursuit, citing the grossly exaggerated "enormity" of loss of life in mitigating his liability for the abandonment of Mochtar. Certainly the most egregious error expressed is Soekarno's tacit acceptance of not only Mochtar's guilt but that of the entire Eijkman Institute. Ordinary Indonesians accepting such claims would view the institute as a thoroughly disgraced enterprise. An outraged Abu Hanifah offered a more blunt assessment of Soekarno:

> My God, either he was just a lamb in Japanese hands or a big dumb liar. But he could have corrected his opinion of 1944 in his book of 1965. He didn't correct the mistake; so he believed in the enormous lie given to him by the murderers of Dr. Muchtar. In doing so, he maintained a story in which one of the best sons of Indonesia has fallen victim to an enormous slander by the Japanese. . . . And in believing the Japanese version of what happened [at Klender] he was guilty of spreading false information and slandering the good name of good sons of Indonesia. This story will also not help Soekarno in convincing people that he acted correctly in the past, especially during the Japanese occupation. Either he was a fool, or just an ignorant man with a tremendous vanity, or worse, a big liar.[4]

Hanifah's unbridled invective illustrates how the truth of Mochtar and the Eijkman Institute entangled and intertwined with the romusha holocaust and Soekarno's dangerous political exposure to it.

The Eijkman Institute had few friends in 1965, and its formal closure was likely met at best with ambivalence. Its death began with the Japanese assigning it responsibility for the calamity at Klender. They pushed it further in that direction by murdering Mochtar. At the end of the Pacific War, the dysfunctional and demoralized Eijkman Institute teetered on collapse. The Dutch war to reestablish its colonial domain over Indonesia, then followed by confrontation over West New Guinea, effectively killed the gravely wounded institute.

The temptation to speculate on a different trajectory for the institute—had the truth at Klender been revealed by a surviving Mochtar or had the Dutch accepted the Republic of Indonesia without conflict—should be resisted as a pointless exercise. History offers no such retries. We need only accept its course and strive to learn from its consequences.

Rebirth

The communist purge beginning in late 1965 launched the New Order regime of Soeharto. Again significantly bloodied, this time by her own hand, impoverished and in social and political tatters, Indonesia had little time or resources for erudite medical research. But that would change.

No matter what historians have to say about tactics during Soeharto's long reign, his strategy certainly led to a strong and stable republic. As Soekarno had done, Soeharto vigorously and ruthlessly suppressed ideologies incompatible with either a secular state or his dominion over it. Islamists in particular suffered oppression and were met with lethal state force when challenging the secular underpinnings of Pancasila and the 1945 constitution. Few outside Indonesia have grasped the depth of its commitment to secular governance. Many in the West, for example, looked upon Soeharto's 1975 invasion of East Timor as simple Islamic hegemony against a Christian enclave. This is demonstrably false and reveals a gross misunderstanding of Indonesian history and national identity that borders upon bigotry.

Soeharto remained concrete and steadfast in the Boedi Oetomo/ Youth Pledge vision of Indonesia Raya, despite his unhealthy appetite for extreme wealth and power. In pursuit of such, however, he laid the foundations for profound economic progress. By 1990 massive foreign investment poured into the stable nation, in large measure because of its enormous potential for economic expansion aided by political stability and broad domestic calm. While the political elite in Jakarta greedily harvested the lion's share of such wealth, a middle class of modest numbers nonetheless emerged. Indonesians were healthier, wealthier, and wiser than ever in their long history to that point.

In that era, an obscure technocrat who had spent most of his adult life in Germany working to help build Airbus Industrie, B. J. Habibie, became Soeharto's minister of science and technology. Habibie launched a variety of technical enterprises, including a modest aircraft manufacturing plant in West Java. Habibie earned a reputation as a technical visionary who got things done by wielding a formidable clout buttressed by reasoned persuasion and personal charm.

In the late 1980s Minister Habibie visited the Institute for Molecular and Cellular Biology (IMCB) at Singapore. He saw that institute for what it was: a Singaporean enterprise aimed at joining and capitalizing on the coming biotechnological revolution. He went directly to President Soeharto for funding for the same in Jakarta. The president complained of having too many roads and bridges to build, but Habibie persisted and prevailed. He positioned his ministry to build a modern biotechnological institute.

In the 1970s Sangkot Marzuki (coauthor) left Jakarta for Australia. He established himself as a tenured professor of molecular medicine at Monash University at Melbourne. He was winning substantial research grants in the realm of mitochondrial biology, and he ran the busiest and most prolific laboratory in his department. In the late 1980s, Sangkot stumbled upon a book in the university library, *Science and Scientists in the Netherlands Indies,* published in 1945 by Dutch war refugees residing in New York. The astonishing scope and quality of scientific research achieved in his native land inspired Marzuki to mobilize recognition of the centenary of Eijkman's 1890 paper linking beriberi to polished rice. He wrote to Habibie.

Minister Habibie did not directly reply to the letter, but he was already beginning the search for an Indonesian scientist to head his new biotechnology institute. In that task he enlisted the help of two of Indonesia's most prominent life scientists. Dr. Pratiwi Sudarmono held a PhD in immunology from Japan and had trained with NASA as an astronaut. The shuttle *Challenger* disaster of 1986 scuttled her lone chance at launch. Dr. A. A. Loedin (who passed away in 2013) was Habibie's choice in leading his search, with Dr. Pratiwi assisting.

Marzuki received a letter from Loedin, innocently inviting him to Jakarta to discuss the future of molecular biology in Indonesia. The visit coincided with the anniversary of Indonesian independence on August 17, and Marzuki was invited to the celebration at the Presidential Palace in Jakarta. Three days later Marzuki met Habibie, reminding him of his proposal to celebrate the work of Christiaan Eijkman and his Nobel Prize, the only one awarded for work done in

Indonesia. Marzuki began a pitch for revitalizing the Eijkman Institute, where that work had been done. Habibie listened, and before Marzuki could finish his appeal, Habibie declared that the old Eijkman Institute building, then near ruin, must be restored to its 1916 grandeur and outfitted as a modern research facility for molecular biology. He enthusiastically committed to that vision on the spot. Ministerial cogs began turning on Habibie's command.

Few of his advisors and ministry officers embraced his concept. Having assessed the old building, they implored him to simply build a new facility at a fraction of the cost. He dismissed this advice, understanding the meaningfulness of history and its lessons. The value of retaining the prestige embedded in the institute's scientific history, Habibie insisted, was priceless. The minister would get what the minister wants, Habibie stubbornly demanded. In 1992, President Soeharto formally opened the reborn Eijkman Institute in a ceremony attended by Minister Habibie and its new director, Professor Marzuki. Also attending was his former student and new deputy, Dr. Hera Sudoyo.

As of late 2013, both remain in these posts. One can marvel at their two decades-long project with a walk through the modern Eijkman Institute for Molecular Biology (Lembaga Biologi Molekular Eijkman). The institute retains, quite deliberately, its early twentieth-century feel. Although its ceilings are still twenty feet high, there is now air-conditioning. Most of the original doors and windows are in place. The elegant original tile floors and marble steps remain, along with stunning original and some replicated stained glass windows depicting a caduceus and chromosomes. The furniture, lighting, and decorations are reproduced or actual antique (many from the original institute), but the laboratories in the massive old building are ultramodern. Through the campaigning of the director and the deputy director, the Eijkman Institute was declared a national historic landmark in 2009 and, as such, will be protected against the exigencies of the intensive latter-day urban development that now surrounds it on all sides.

Parking spaces at the enormous hospital adjacent to the institute are too few, and an undignified, jarringly modern sea of hundreds of motorbikes substitutes for a grass lawn at the institute's facade.

The building's spacious courtyard provides staff parking between a central fountain and a garden fringe, giving the impression of peaceful solitude in a secret haven (idle automobiles notwithstanding).

The beauty of the reborn Eijkman Institute runs deeper than eye-pleasing architecture and gardens. As it did in the late nineteenth century, when it was called the Central Laboratory for Public Health, and in the early twentieth century, after it was named in honor of Christiaan Eijkman, the institute stands as an oasis of science and the culture that supports it. That culture is the intellectual pursuit of the bald truth—one often very hard to decipher and inconvenient to accept—in other words, the hard core of science.

Habibie insulated the Eijkman Institute from bureaucratic jockeying and politics, creating a semiautonomous entity largely free of stifling regulations and constraints. Technical merit and competitiveness, Habibie understood, drives the scientific enterprise. Science is blind to bureaucratic titles and careers, seeing only merit in new understanding and in those who provide it. Science is also ambivalent to the pride and vanity we attach to its successful execution. Admiration of brilliance and accomplishment is embedded in our human nature, and we treasure institutions that permit their expression and the ongoing march of human progress. The Eijkman Institute did so in the past, and its scientists relish and nurtur its potential to continue doing so in the future.

Ghosts

The restored Eijkman Institute building looks essentially as it did in 1941, save the subdued intrusions of air-conditioning, a bio-safety level 3 laboratory consuming a bit of the courtyard, and a tower erected to overcome the blockage of digital signal reception by an adjacent hospital high-rise. Those new constructions are period perfect, as if built in 1916. The signature Dutch colonial tunnel entrance at the front and center of the institute, where the Kenpeitai man in civilian clothing awaited the unsuspecting Hanafiah on his bicycle, remains the only means of entering the institute.

The furnishings in common areas are also to period, and one finds a scattering of pieces clearly identifiable in photographs within the institute during the 1930s. One of those photos shows W. K. Mertens, the director, sitting at his desk, presumably the same one Mochtar would later use. That desk now sits in a suite near the deputy director's office. The bookcases shown behind Mertens at work now reside in a conference room off the institute's auditorium. These and other fine pieces were somehow not lost during the forty-seven-year quiescence of the institute.

Where once stood the library of the old Eijkman Institute—where Kenpeitai thugs assembled Hanafiah and his colleagues for arrest—now hangs a large portrait of Achmad Mochtar. It is a contemporary pastel, commissioned from the photograph of Achmad and his wife, Siti Hasnah, ca. 1927. It joins portraits of Eijkman and his colleague Grijns in a foyer before the director's suite. The confident smile of Mochtar is captured as in the original photo. His portrait gazes over the comings and goings of young and old scientists, Indonesians and their foreign collaborators who are charged with the energy of the pursuit of understanding and knowledge of biology and medicine. The physical institute and the human spirit residing within it would be immediately recognizable to Mochtar.

In late December 1944, Mochtar whispered comfort to a fellow prisoner scientist at the Jakarta Kenpeitai prison: "All is fine now." At long last, it is.

Epilogue

Cimahi

Just to the west of Bandung lies the community of Cimahi. It is pronounced "chee mah hee." Using pre-1950 spelling dominated by Dutch phonetics, it is Tjimahi, as Ancol was Antjol or "ahn chole." The climate is more agreeable in this mountainous region, cooler and less humid than Jakarta. Weekenders stream out of Jakarta using the new toll road that cuts the trip from six hours to just two. Residents of Bandung complain they must stay home on weekends because the heavy traffic makes navigating their city unbearable. Outlet malls, local cuisine, the climate, and the city's progressive social atmosphere prove irresistible to Jakarta's swelling middle class. Pleasant forested hills loom nearby Cimahi. But these fine surroundings belie the hell that occurred at this place during the Pacific War. This was the site of a large internment camp for Dutch civilians operated by the Japanese.

The modern highway exit sign from the Jakarta toll road, at the western edge of metropolitan Bandung, reads "Cimahi" and "Pasteur." Taking that exit, one may further follow the signs to Leuwigajah to the west for a kilometer or so. A broken and crowded road brings one to a large Chinese cemetery on the left. At the cemetery gate, some eighty or so meters within the grounds, an alert visitor may spot a large black forged iron gate with "Ereveld" written in gold across its top. This is the cemetery maintained by a Dutch-Indonesian foundation (the same one that manages Ancol) to hold the remains of the thousands who did not survive the harsh captivity at Cimahi.

The malignant and willful neglect of these captives killed as surely as any executioner's sword. Tombstones at the Cimahi cemetery for the obliquely murdered substantially outnumber those for the forthrightly murdered at Ancol.

There are the remains of others, too. A scattering of graves bear post–August 1945 dates, memorializing people who perished in the war of independence. Virtually all of these are the Indonesian names of KNIL (by then called NICA, the Netherlands Indies Civil Administration) soldiers who fought against their countrymen. Among them are Muslim and Christian grave markers. These men remained loyal to the Dutch and made the ultimate sacrifice for them. They were brought here to rest among those to whom their loyalties remained steadfast. This was not vindictive but sensible and humane.

To the far right of the Ereveld and about forty rows deep from the east is the Christian grave marked "W. K. Mertens," with a date of death of February 21, 1945. Dr. Mertens had been the director of the Eijkman Institute before Mochtar. Born at Surabaya, Mertens was a son of the archipelago but also a Dutchman. He likely would not have ascribed to the racial apartheid of his colonial countrymen. The institute he directed was the antithesis of such. This internment camp or others like it were home, as he knew it, in his last three years of life: a harsh and bitter apartheid imposed upon the whites of Java by the Japanese occupier.

We know the Kenpeitai brought Mertens to Jakarta to serve as an expert witness in the investigation of the Klender event. Several Eijkman staff in Kenpeitai captivity later described seeing him at the prison on Koningsplien, along with Professor Dinger. All of them recalled that Mertens was too ill to speak, and the physician Hanafiah and technician Jatman each explicitly described him as suffering advanced beriberi. His lower legs and feet were grotesquely swollen—a classical sign of that malady. The terrible unremitting pain took away his ability to speak. With awful irony, the man who directed the institute that had provided certain knowledge of the cause, prevention, and cure of beriberi suffered that painful and protracted death. Mertens had plenty of company in this misery at Cimahi; beriberi killed tens of inmates on a daily basis as the cruel chronic starvation among the captives firmed its grip.

Dr. Otten, the former director of the nearby Pasteur Institute, may have attended Mertens. He was also interred at Cimahi, and these former Eijkman colleagues surely visited one another during their years in captivity. Dr. Otten survived the camp and was repatriated to Holland, but he died on November 7, 1946, a few weeks after his return. Today, in downtown Bandung, a crowded and lively street named "Jalan Dr. Otten" leads to the main hospital, Rumah Sakit Hasan Sadikin. Otten is remembered as the man who brought prominence to the Pasteur Institute at Bandung with its groundbreaking work on crucial vaccines. These people at Bandung, who the Japanese discarded into the hell of Cimahi, likely bear responsibility for sparing millions of lives with their superb vaccines. The institute they built continues doing so today.

Ancol

On June 2, 2010, we left the Eijkman Institute at Salemba and drove the few miles to the Ereveld at Ancol in North Jakarta. It is tricky to find. One must enter the vast seaside amusement compound of Dunia Fantasi (Fantasy World) and pay the modest fee for doing so. The friendly people collecting the fee do not indulge requests for fee exemption from those wanting only to visit the cemetery. Sticking close to the seafront and driving in an easterly direction, eventually one stumbles upon the large wrought iron gates of the Ereveld. The lonely keepers are welcoming, always happy to see visitors.

The cemetery sits on the shore of the Java Sea. The sea is gentle here. Waves do not crash at Ancol but quietly lap. Significant earthworks had recently been completed to protect the cemetery from the rare flooding that had threatened it. A four-meter-high berm blocks the ocean view along its length. In July 1945, the view of the sea would have been unobstructed.

The amusement park surrounds the cemetery on its three landward sides, but it is a relatively quiet nook. There are a few seaside restaurants nearby, but none of the roller-coaster rumbles, carnival music, screaming, and laughing that fills the air of the park a kilometer or so to the west.

On westward approach to Soekarno-Hatta International Airport, airplanes fly at a couple of thousand feet over the sea along the Jakarta waterfront. The cemetery is plainly visible to those who know where to look, just west of the prominent wharfs of the busy Tanjung Priok port. The cemetery ground is an imperfect tapering rectangular plot about 250 meters long and maybe 100 at its widest. Once inside the large compound of the cemetery, all is quiet. The berm and a fringe of thick trees and its immaculately landscaped grounds give it the feel of a secluded sanctuary.

In 1945 all here was isolated natural marshland, far from the bustle of old Jakarta. The execution ground was a hidden piece of Japanese occupation ugliness. At a remote Buddhist temple somewhere nearby, a deaf and mute caretaker lived like a hermit. At war's end he approached the Allied authorities and communicated to them what he had been witnessing at the marsh since 1942: Japanese soldiers routinely beheading people at a tree near the seafront. He brought them to the ghastly mound of earth emanating the stench of death. He pointed out the tree.

We carried a printed copy of an email from Iris Heidebrink at the Netherlands War Archive (NIOD) in Amsterdam that, to our astonishment, seemed to pinpoint the location of the grave of Mochtar at Ereveld Ancol. On the Indonesian side up to that point, all accounts of his execution and burial had left us almost without hope of locating his remains. The notes described only a mass grave or rubbish heap near the sea as the place where the Japanese disposed of his body. No one, at least in Indonesia, seemed to be aware that his burial site was known. Those who would have cared the most in 1946, had they tried to locate Mochtar's grave, would have faced the formidable barrier of approaching a very busy and militarily belligerent new government. Iris's 2010 email came as a thunderbolt of revelation.

In Hanafiah's booklet on the Mochtar affair, published in 1976, he described the dead end he reached in trying to find where Mochtar had been buried. The Japanese officers he approached after the surrender simply shrugged. However, his privately published autobiography of 1977 tells of finding and visiting the grave of Mochtar at the same location identified by the Dutch archivists. He wrote again of having had no hope of ever finding it, but on November 20, 1976, at the urging of a friend, he went to the cemetery at Ancol and found the placard bearing the name of his beloved brother-in-law and colleague.[1]

In June 2010, not yet aware of Hanafiah's autobiography and discovery thirty-four years earlier, we arrived at the cemetery at 3 p.m., unsure of what might be found. According to Hanafiah's memoir, citing no sources for his information, Mochtar had been executed on the site at 3 p.m. on July 13, 1945. The Dutch records, taken from a Japanese log of executions at the Ancol site, put his death on July 3, 1945. If we accept the 3 p.m. time, it would have been very warm and humid, as it was during our first exploration of the cemetery. The sun was approaching the westerly horizon in clear skies, just beginning to color the sea in reddish orange hues.

Most of the tombstones marked the burial site of the unknown remains excavated from the mass grave. However, lists of names appeared on many placards placed among those tombstones. They appeared to list alphabetically the names of those known to have been executed at Ancol—that list recovered from Japanese records by the returning Allies. After some confusion and wandering about the grounds, Professor Sangkot found the marker and hailed its location. It was a quiet and contemplative moment. We didn't speak. Professor Mochtar's name was inscribed with nine others on a single placard placed between tombstones that read in Dutch "Executed at Ancol." That placard spoke across the sixty-five years, "Here is where they put me."

With the exception of his dear friend and fellow prisoner Hanafiah in 1976, Mochtar had had no known friendly visitors since the moment of his abduction from his home by the Kenpeitai on Saturday, October 7, 1944. Soon, though, the martyred Achmad Mochtar would be welcomed back into the warm bosom of his family, his colleagues, and his nation.

Family

After accepting his death, Mochtar's large extended family mourned his passing, but had no certain knowledge of his death or where his remains lay at rest. At war's end, Siti Hasnah regained possession of her home, Hastarimba, at Jalan Raden Saleh No. 48. She would remain there until her death in 1963. A photograph of her from around 1960 shows a silver-haired and bespectacled Siti Hasnah in a fine Javanese batik sarong and kebaya blouse (fig. 36). She gazes directly into the camera, as in the 1927 portrait with Mochtar. Her expression is neither happiness nor sadness. She stands alone wearing the festive outfit. She appears lonely. Siti Hasnah's remains are buried at the large cemetery at Karet not far from the Shangri-La Hotel in central Jakarta. Mochtar's nephew, Abu Hanifah, lies in the same cemetery. He passed away at Gatot Subroto Army Hospital in January 1980, honored as a hero of the republic.

Siti Hasnah's son Imramsjah survived the war in Europe and returned home in March 1947, bringing his sweetheart from Leiden, Marie Antoinette Lancel, twenty-six years old. In 2010 Asikin Hanafiah recalled that Imramsjah's mother had sent him off to Holland with one simple and very firm admonishment: "Do not marry a Dutch woman over there." A defensive Imramsjah explained to his irate mother that he had obeyed her order. He did not marry a Dutch woman over there, but intended to marry her in Indonesia. Siti Hasnah at first refused to bless the union. Imramsjah reluctantly accepted his mother's protests, recalled Asikin, and then asserted, "Then I shall never marry." Siti Hasnah relented, blessed them, and they married in Jakarta on March 28 of that year.

Dr. Imramsjah Mochtar returned to Amsterdam in 1951 for postgraduate studies at the University of Amsterdam and completed those in 1954 as his father had done in 1926 and his daughter, Monique, would do in 2011. He returned to Indonesia and settled briefly in Surabaya in 1955, but Imramsjah and Marie returned to Amsterdam for good in 1958. The Mochtars of Amsterdam had two daughters, Astrid Jolanda Mochtar, born in Jakarta in 1949, and Monique Hasnah Mochtar, born in 1961 in Amsterdam. Marie Lancel had a son from a previous marriage, Bujono Purnomohadi, who was born in Amsterdam. Imramsjah adopted him.

Monique explained that everyone called her father "De" (pronounced "Day"), after his middle name, Ade. In 2010 both Jolanda and Monique recalled several visits to their childhood home in Amsterdam by the old family friend, Abu Hanifah. Dr. Hanifah had risen to prominence in the new government of Indonesia. This STOVIA graduate had been a Youth Pledge leader, physician, nationalist politician, and then commander of an armed commando unit in West Java during the war of independence—a hero of the republic. After being the first minister of education, science, and culture, he was posted to Brazil and to Italy as ambassador. He would also lead the Indonesian UNICEF delegation at the United Nations in New York. The women remembered Oom Abu as very soft-spoken with long, elegant fingers and as the reliable bearer of gifts for little girls. Jolanda holds a manuscript written by Hanifah. He had handed it over to De for safekeeping. Stormy Indonesia of the 1960s consumed some critical writers and thinkers, and Hanifah had explained that the work contained material many in government would find disturbing. It is perhaps an early draft of his *Tales of a Revolution*, which indeed would have inspired consternation among Soekarno loyalists of that dangerous era. Hanifah could not remain silent on the brutality of the Japanese occupation. He demanded acknowledgment of the romusha holocaust.

Jolanda, who left Indonesia with her parents in 1958 at age nine, recalled the unhappy circumstances of departing. She winced slightly when she remembered graffiti painted on their home in Surabaya that read "anjing Belanda" (Dutch dog). Hostility toward the Dutch over possession of what the Indonesians claimed as Irian Jaya, Dutch New Guinea, festered at this time. Jolanda remembered her father later explaining that he had been sickened by the corruption he encountered in the new republic. An assault on Marie's car by an angry mob at Surabaya was simply the last straw. The family retreated to Holland for good.

In 2010 Asikin Hanafiah recalled De coming out to Schiphol airport at Amsterdam to sit with him as he transited to London for medical training in the 1960s. They sat and discussed news and the old days in Jakarta. The kindness and gentle demeanor of the aging De very much reminded Asikin of his uncle Achmad. Dr. Imramsjah Mochtar became professor of medicine, specializing in pediatric hematology at the University of Amsterdam. He published more than fifty peer-reviewed journal articles. He went on to discover several of the dozen or so known human clotting factors. He died suddenly on April 18, 1980, when he was just sixty-two. His loving family bid him farewell at his cremation at Westgaarde in Amsterdam.

Imramsjah's father never had a farewell. The Japanese abducted him, tortured him, took his life, and tossed his remains onto the pile of bones and rotting flesh of the hundreds of others they had murdered. They jotted down his particulars in their book of the murdered and walked away.

"We Shall Remember Them"

The staff of the modern Eijkman Institute, upon learning with certainty of Mochtar's remains resting at the Ancol cemetery, resolved to right that wrong. Sangkot Marzuki and Hera Sudoyo, director and deputy director, planned and orchestrated a memorial service for Mochtar on the sixty-fifth anniversary of his loss, Saturday, July 3, 2010.

After much reflection, Sangkot decided that a dawn service would be most fitting. The poem on the awful tree at Ancol closes with "And in the morning, we shall remember them, we shall remember them." Doing so seemed fitting and proper. The service aimed at celebrating the life of Mochtar rather than the darkness of his death. Not knowing with certainty the time of his execution, Sangkot aimed at celebrating the anniversary of Mochtar's last few hours of life.

Just five days before that ceremony, contact had been established for the first time with Mochtar's surviving granddaughters in Holland, Jolanda van der Bom and Dr. Monique Hasnah Mochtar. Staff at the Netherlands War Archive had approached them, asking if they wished to be contacted on this matter. They did. They learned of the planned ceremony. Jolanda immediately instructed her son, Mochtar's great-grandson Michiel Gerard, living in Kuala Lumpur, Malaysia, to attend on behalf of the family. A day later, she and her husband, Martijn, and other son, Martijn John (who in the coming year would legally add Imramsjah to the front of his given name), decided they must also attend. The entire van der Bom clan departed for Jakarta. And finally, with just four hours to go before being able to catch the last connection to Jakarta, Monique also decided that she had to attend. She made the mad dash to Schiphol.

All of Mochtar's family from Holland (and Malaysia) managed to arrive in Jakarta the day before the ceremony. We gathered with them for dinner at the expansive and elegant home of Dr. Asikin Hanafiah at Pejaten Barat in south Jakarta. Jolanda and Monique recalled learning of what had happened to their grandfather in a Dutch newspaper article in 1983, three years after their father had passed away. He had never spoken of it and rarely spoke of his father at all. Only later did they understand what dreadful pain the memory of his father's execution must have caused. The dawn ceremony was deliberately low-key and solemn, with about fifty invited guests attending. All wore khaki pants and white shirts and were each issued a red bandana for the neck or arm—a symbol of patriotic mourning. The people who cared most about Mochtar and his life were all present, with the exception of his daughter-in-law, Marie Lancel, who was nearly ninety and too frail to journey from Holland. His dear niece Taty also could not attend—the precipitous nature of the ceremony caught her out of town. Nephew Asikin Hanafiah and his wife were present. Latifah Marzoeki and her son Arjito appeared as well. The senior scientists from Eijkman were all present, along with many of the younger scientists and students, serving to have things run smoothly but also learning of a rich and tragic piece of their institutional history.

The people gathered under a pavilion where a large portrait of Mochtar stood, the one normally found hanging at the entrance to the director's suite. The feeling of the old Eijkman Institute—strong and friendly Dutch-Indonesian bonds, indifference to racial identity, and the spirit of apolitical scientific excellence—breathed to life in that cemetery. Could Mochtar have seen, he would have looked upon his Dutch granddaughters and great-grandsons, his loving nephew, Asikin, the daughter of his friend Marzoeki, Latifah, and the proud new Indonesian Eijkman Institute scientists. He would have smiled in firm and familiar recognition. These were his people and his legacy, his family of kin and kindred gathered to remember and honor him.

Sangkot called this gathering from coffee and chatting at 6 a.m., as the unseen sun rose behind low overcast and threat of rain. His remarks were friendly and informal, as Mochtar himself would have been. He moved us to the site of the placard where Mochtar's name appears. A smaller portrait of Mochtar leaned against it. Sangkot again spoke, reminding those present of Mochtar's life and of his sacrifice. Flowers were laid by all present, one by one. As a light sprinkle began, a string quartet of Eijkman scientists played "Gugur Bunga Taman Bakti" (The fallen flower in the garden of devotion) composed by Ismail Marzuki for those who lost their lives in the struggle for independence. The lyrics inspire:

How can I not feel sorrow
My hero has passed
How can I not feel sad
I am left all alone

Who can be my solace
Loyal and brave
Who can be my heart's hero
A true defender of the people

My hero has passed
His service is done
One falls, a thousand arise
For our great and sacred homeland

My flower has fallen in the garden of devotion
On our mother's lap
The fragrance pervades the essence
Of our great and sacred homeland

Umbrellas appeared. Asikin Hanafiah delivered a prayer for Mochtar. Georgina Tapiheru, a young scientist at the Eijkman, picked up her guitar and sang a soulful rendering of "Tanah Airku" (My land and seas)—not the national anthem, but to Indonesians very much like "America the Beautiful" is to Americans in its national inspirational quality. The service concluded with the string quartet playing a mournfully patriotic "Bagimu Negeri." Distant passersby stopped and stared at these goings-on in the normally deserted cemetery. Someone long dead but still remembered is being honored today, they would have realized.

Responsibility

This book offers what we know about Mochtar and the events that put him under that tree at Ancol in 1945. The case for the Japanese experiment at Klender remains circumstantial in 2014. "Circumstantial," though it is a qualifying term, should not be misconstrued as unreliable or even unproven. It simply means a lack of direct proof. If a man wakes in the morning to find a fresh blanket of snow on his lawn under clear skies, he draws the conclusion that there had been a snowfall while he slept. He did not see it snowing, but he sees its aftermath and knows that falling snow rationally explains the circumstantial evidence before him.[2] This book examines the blanket of snow left by the Mochtar affair and builds an argument that rationally explains what occurred.

A parallel with circumstantial evidence in criminal prosecution may be drawn. The strength of evidence-driven reason and rationality of an incriminating explanation may be sufficient for considering a case proven beyond reasonable doubt. If, however, the accused presents an exculpatory explanation of equal or greater reason and rationality accounting for how the incriminating evidence misleads, the circumstantial evidence-based case crumbles. Absent such, conviction ensues. No person or government has come forward with an explanation of the Klender event that aligns better or as well with the known facts as that posed in this book. Silence in the face of this incriminating argument would affirm the veracity of its logical conclusion.

An imagined counsel for the defense of the Japanese army men at Bandung would surely point to the weakness of the direct evidence. No record exists of the romusha at Klender being given the prime and boost vaccinations that must have occurred if the hypothesized experiment, challenge with pure tetanus toxin, in fact took place. No documentation or testimony from the Pasteur Institute proves the Japanese were in pursuit of a toxoid vaccine like their navy counterparts at Surabaya. No testimony or document places the Japanese vaccine makers from Bandung at the Klender camp in the weeks leading up to the event. No record of Japanese high command or Kenpeitai deliberation of the event at Klender is known, much less their decision-making in its wake. The imagined counsel would ask for acquittal on these grounds. Counsel would not mention that the records at the Pasteur Institute had been destroyed by the Japanese.[3]

The rational counter to that argument is relatively simple and direct—there is no doubt regarding the presence of lethal amounts of tetanus toxin in the vaccinations administered at Klender, and the only rational explanation of this fact that aligns with all of the available evidence is an experiment, like the one at Surabaya. A failed experiment rationally accounts for the event and all of the available direct evidence, as well as Japanese actions in the Mochtar affair. We can think of no other scenario grounded in reason that could do so, nor has one been offered.

The Imperial Japanese Army and Navy men in occupied Indonesia behaved as monstrously as they did elsewhere in their conquered lands. They invaded Indonesia with the intent of colonial imperial domination. The Japanese revision of this truth began in the months leading to their defeat, when they finally acted on one of the many deceptions of their occupation: independence for Indonesia. The bald truth of the enslavement, torture, rape, and murder of Indonesians was concealed under domestic and international political wraps. Those wraps continue serving Japanese nationalists in their efforts to market the deception of noble intent and behavior by their armed forces during the Pacific War.

Lessons

The Pacific War destroyed many institutions and ways of life, and good riddance to those like colonial imperialism, militarism, and fascism. The new independent nations all across the region—Indonesia, Malaysia, Singapore, Myanmar, Cambodia, Laos, Vietnam, China, Taiwan, South Korea, and the Philippines—would later ignite the revolution of development and progress (a march of progress led by reconstructed Japan) that drives the global economy. But war pays no such dividends. The cooperative and productive behavior of the survivors of war does.

The yield of warfare between peoples never deviates from its core deliverables—rapacious and cruel self-interest, stinking death, and the raw elements of human misery: fear, hunger, pain, sorrow, and hopelessness. The people of Indonesia thus suffered during their occupation by Imperial Japan, a brutal invader that the colonial masters of the region had arrogantly underestimated and ineptly failed to repel. The colonialists had lorded over their domains with a complex mix of genuine beneficence and greed, but the catastrophic failure to protect those residing within them engendered the moral grounds for terminating the colonial enterprise. The shameless attempt to reassert Holland's colonial reign in the wake of that failure wreaked further damage upon Indonesians and the trajectory of their new republic. Indonesians bore heavy costs for their long colonization, the Pacific War, and the cruel struggle for independence that followed it.

The long silent injustice of the Mochtar affair was one such cost. Political exigencies gave shelter to those responsible for his murder and uncounted others. Barbaric Imperial Japanese behavior and the pursuit of its truth became inconvenient, embarrassing, and threatening to political leaders in Indonesia during and after the war of independence. Domestic political risk to the collaborating nationalists eased by sliding the weight of national historic emphasis away from Japanese brutality and toward nobility. The Dutch return after the Pacific War not only buttressed that deception but also made it necessary in defense of the new republic. Those events eased the Japanese task of refashioning their motivations into the noble ideal of a free Indonesia.

Other events further encouraged Japanese wishful thinking on the nobility of their war. The Americans insulated the emperor of Japan, Hirohito, from war tribunal proceedings—a lone exception among Axis leaders. Many hundreds of Japanese soldiers arrested soon after the war for murder were later released without trial because their victims were not prisoners of war. The complete personal liberty granted the Unit 731 criminals without even arrest has been detailed. Finally, the release of all convicted Japanese war criminals from prison in 1958 seemed to affirm the Japanese view, then and now, that the Allied tribunals were a sham and their military men had not actually behaved criminally.

Moral Conflict

Whereas Hitler and his Nazis were justly assigned to the rubbish bin of humanity, Imperial Japan somehow got a pass. They had been in formal alliance with the Nazis, shared their brutish worldview, and behaved as monstrously. But the management of justice between them stands as starkly distinct as black and white or, more to the point, evil versus good. Up to the present day the American and German governments assiduously pursue Nazis who evaded justice seventy years ago. In June 2014 an eighty-nine-year-old naturalized American citizen, Hans Breyer, was jailed and held without bail awaiting arraignment for the allegation that, as a teenager, he served as a Waffen ss guard at Auschwitz. Dozens of such cases of former Nazis brought to justice have occurred over the decades, but not a single Japanese soldier has been arrested and tried since the last Pacific War tribunal hearing in 1956. Consider the 2002 bbc interview of Unit 731 veteran Toshimi Mizobuchi and his frank admission, without remorse then or now, of killing many Chinese prisoners in medical experiments. He spoke freely, without fear of being held to account. No one would bring him to justice, as he certainly understood.

What accounts for such indifferent lassitude concerning Japanese war criminals versus the abiding pursuit of justice against the Nazis? Rationally reconciling those treatments would require invoking a great moral distance between the wartime conduct of the Imperial Japanese and the Nazis, such as good versus evil. In this light the Japanese could be forgiven for believing they were indeed a very different enemy from the Nazis, that is, neither criminally militaristic nor inhumane. But they were both. Another possible explanation of this conflict, then, is a moral failure by the managers of that justice. Does selfish national reward motivate the leniency and amnesia regarding Japanese behavior in the war?

Japan and South Korea represent the strategic lynchpins of American presence and influence in the region, both economic and military. The U.S. relationship to each is extraordinarily friendly, prosperous, and genuinely valued. These nations today are remarkably like-minded and integrated despite the vast geographic, historic, and cultural distances between them. Though national friends like the United States and the United Kingdom, in contrast, share much, many Americans would view South Korea and Japan as warmly as Great Britain. Immigration and large prosperous and influential Korean and Japanese American communities in part explain this genuine warmth. So too does the deliberately cultivated social blindness to racial identity aspired to by the Americans. The United States has deep interests in East Asia—historic, social, political, and economic. The U.S. desire to protect those interests is as legitimate as it is important.

China and North Korea, each in their own way, resent and fear those friendships. This has dominated the strategic equation for East Asia for the past seventy years. The American government, despite recent threat-inspired attention on the Middle East, has never faltered in its commitment to East Asian friends. In addition to the Pacific War itself, the Americans fought two other costly wars protecting those interests and friends, one to stalemate (Korea) and the other to defeat (Vietnam). The economic rise of the region and its importance to American economic vigor deepens that commitment today. Confronting valued Japanese friends on their view of a long-ago war perhaps seems inexpedient and rash, all very heavy things and costs considered.

These considerations, it seems, efface moral clarity on a grave injustice. French Algerian Nobel laureate Albert Camus wrote, "In such a world of conflict, a world of victims and executioners, it is the job of thinking people not to be on the side of executioners."[4] The actions of the American government with regard to management of justice for the victims of Imperial Japan, especially in the harsh light of that delivered against Nazi criminals, begs critical reflection. How did justice for the victims of Imperial Japanese brutality become so freely disposable and utterly forgotten? How did the injustice of honoring their executioners become acceptable behavior in a valued ally and friend?

Truth in politics may be mutable and negotiable, but no deceit eradicates it. Vaporous conjured truths rarely outlast the granite of the real truth they conceal and its consequences. The people bearing the burden of an injustice will seek to right what is wrong.

Injustice

Conservative Japanese nationalists turn the enabling strategic situation to their advantage when proffering their version of Japan's history in the Pacific War. Some have become aggressively revisionist, duplicitously erasing grotesque misdeeds of enormous scale from the pages of Japan's history and honoring the memories of the mass murderers and rapists who carried out those crimes. The lives lost among their neighbors, the revisionists espouse, were victims of the American and European colonial imperialists (and their Chinese allies) who made war against a Japanese nation striving to liberate their bullied fellow Asians. Even worse, the victimized nations of their Pacific War, they imply, were the beneficiaries of their ultimately successful campaign against the blue-eyed colonial imperialists, as in Indonesia. It is akin to the absurd idea that the nation of Israel was a gift born of Nazi sacrifice. When the government of China expresses outrage at Japan's reinvention of the causes, motivations, conduct, and outcome of World War II, it refers to these historically and morally corrupt notions.

The revisionist Japanese nationalists crave the delusional certainty that their soldiers and sailors brought no dishonor to their nation. In leveraging the liberty to mutate history granted by the principal victor of the Pacific War muted on this subject, the revisionists apply what drove them to become a conquered nation in first place—naked and vainly selfish nationalism standing upon the make-believe nobility of their Pacific War.

The grave consequences of such deep injustice may be seen in the seas and air spaces bordering Japan, China, and the Korean Peninsula in December 2013. American, South Korean, and Japanese warplanes defy Chinese unilateral assertion of an air defense identification zone (ADIZ) over a vast swath of ocean. Chinese eyes see an unrepentant Japan aided and abetted by Americans laying claim to Chinese territory. They aim to upset that claim and rationally argue that Japan and South Korea administer their own unilaterally established ADIZS (not citing the relatively very modest sizes of those zones). Japanese and American eyes, on the other hand, see the vast China ADIZ as a precipitous and dangerous element of a resurgent militarism in the sphere by a rising and arming China. It is an irksome challenge to a seventy-year status quo. China, in turn, engenders such wariness by their reliance on displays of military muscle in managing other contested maritime claims rather than equitable compromise with its neighbors. The underlying organic national passions impose a hair-trigger for military clash.

At the roots of this very dangerous posturing is the profound injustice of the unacknowledged, denied, and erased crimes committed by the Japanese armed forces during the Pacific War. According to Jane Perlez writing on the front page of the *International New York Times* on December 4, 2013, the president of China, Xi Jinping—in an impromptu encounter with Japanese prime minister Shinzo Abe in St. Petersburg, Russia, in September 2013—curtly told Abe that Japan must face "history squarely." In that rare spontaneous moment, the head of state spoke to his counterpart not of territorial integrity but of historical integrity. This perhaps glimpses Chinese primacy of reasoning regarding the dangerous tension in their relationship with Japan.

Construing the genuine outrage of China against Japanese revision of a crucial shared history as a disingenuous means of seeking strategic advantage is both gratuitously cynical and exceedingly dangerous. The epic suffering of China under a Japanese invader and occupier merits Chinese outrage at attempts to expunge it from the records. Extremely selfish national vanity coldly denies and systematically edits that history with American assent by silence on one side, and the other engages in angry and prideful provocations. In these self-serving postures, each of the three principal nations involved court real catastrophe for all of humanity.

The emergent and powerful Chinese will not and should not capitulate to the Japanese nationalist whitewash of their brutalization at the hands of the Imperial Japanese army. The Japanese nationalists today apply that veneer with ever more verve and audacity, buoyed by a sympathetic government expressing and acting in line with their selfish aspirations. American acquiescence to Japan's revisionist behavior deepens the hatreds of the region born of the Pacific War and amplifies risk of the military crises they earnestly seek to avert. Justice heals as effectively as injustice injures—delivering one or the other ordains the results of doing so.

Legacy

Mochtar's treatment by the Japanese echoes their far broader actions during and after the Pacific War. They acted deliberately in concealing the truth of their inhumanity by deflection of blame for the calamitous consequences of their selfish actions. As they put Mochtar forth as the killer of the romusha at Klender, they proffer European colonial imperialist aggression as having caused the Pacific War. Their enemies defeated the noble causes of vaccinating the romusha supporting their war efforts and, in the broader context, of liberating their fellow Asians from the exploitive imperialists. Real motivations belie each of those deceits—a cruel medical experiment on valueless human beings and ruthlessly establishing their own colonial dominion over all of Asia and its "black slaves." These truths, shameful and dangerous, should be considered and managed as verified. Society tolerating denial and deflection of blame for the murders of Mochtar, the romusha, and many other millions in the cause of a racist and fascist ideology deeply degrades our collective humanity. Intolerance of such yields a powerful counter that protects us from a future of darkness—justice grounded in verified, immutable, and nonnegotiable truth.

Mochtar pitted courage and selflessness against the cowardice and selfishness of his tormentors. His moral triumph was not a product of being an extraordinary Indonesian, Muslim, or scientist, but of being an exemplary human being who happened to be all those things. We are more than our inborn, assigned, or selected group identities; we are members of humanity, and the sum of our individual actions toward others defines the collective human experience. The evil among us utterly disregard the happiness and well-being of others. The truly good among us, as Mochtar demonstrated, embrace the happiness and well-being of others as an intrinsic and unshakable human duty, even when doing so comes at tremendous pain and sacrifice.

Mochtar's legacy is the highest expression of personal selflessness in answer to the most extreme selfishness. In revealing the true nature of both in this history, we find the stark lessons of the best and worst of our inner lights as living beings. The capacity for each resides within all of us. The responses of Mochtar and his captors to their events teach us that we are the authors of our own human goodness or evil, as ultimately defined by how our actions impact others. The fate of humanity, either to suffer dark misery or to enjoy bright happiness, hinges upon our choice between selfish harm or selfless succor. Mochtar's story offers testimony of the power of that choice and its consequences.

APPENDIX

Notes on Indonesian Language

Bahasa Indonesia is a formal language with rules and structures like any other. It is, however, the first language of relatively few Indonesians. The mother tongue of most Indonesians is that of their island and group of origin or heritage. Take the examples of the adjacent islands of Java, Bali, and Lombok. Most people on Java speak either Javanese (in the east and center) or Sundanese (in the west). These complex Sanskrit-based languages (and alphabets) share a few words but little else with bahasa Indonesia. One fluent in bahasa Indonesia often finds Javanese or Sundanese incomprehensible. The same is true of bahasa Bali, and fluency in Javanese does not provide a functional grasp of Balinese language. Indonesians on the island of Lombok speak bahasa Sasak, and this language too is incomprehensible to native Javanese and Balinese speakers. Indonesians from all across their vast archipelago use bahasa Indonesia not only as a convenient lingua franca but also as a vital dimension of their identity and unity as a nation. Bahasa Indonesia is the compulsory language of state schools, government, commerce, and media. Virtually all Indonesians are fluent in this language, second to hundreds of mother tongues across the archipelago.

The phonetics of bahasa Indonesia are much simpler than in English, with its many oddities and exceptions. Words are pronounced as spelled and lack varieties of possessive, tense, or masculine/feminine. It uses the same twenty-six letter alphabet, and all consonants are pronounced as in English with one exception: the letter *c* is pronounced as the *ch* in English phonetics. The vowels are pronounced differently, e.g., the *i* sounds like the English *e*. Much of the difficult grammar of a proper English sentence is absent, but conjunctions of root words using a wide range of prefixes and suffixes provide structure and meaning. While functional bahasa Indonesia is acquired with relative ease, genuine fluency is as difficult and laborious as any foreign language.

The origins of bahasa Indonesia reach back long before the colonial era, though one finds borrowed words from the Dutch, English, Spanish, and Portuguese. The language also uses Hindi, Arabic, Japanese, and Chinese words. Trade with Hindi-speaking Indians may have begun as early as the first century. Vibrant and frequent trade was likely underway in the early second millennium. Arab trade with the Sumatran Hindu Srivijaya kingdom likely commenced around 900 AD. The famous Chinese admiral Zheng He frequented the Malacca straits and Java in the early 1400s. An informal lingua franca emerged over the millennia, but it is firmly rooted in the language of the Srivijaya dynasty, which reached across the Malacca straits to today's peninsular Malaysia. Philippine Tagalog also derives from this language.

The STOVIA medical students and the Youth Pledge authors described in this history deliberately made the link between that lingua franca and nationalism. Though all were fluent in Dutch as well as their assorted mother tongues, they preferred their lingua franca when speaking among themselves. After the Youth Pledge of 1928, Indonesian scholars began laying out the formal rules of bahasa Indonesia. The Republic of Indonesia declared bahasa Indonesia a formal language upon national independence in 1945.

Dutch phonetics had strongly influenced the spelling of early standards for bahasa Indonesia in Latin script. For example, the sound of the letter *j* was represented by *dj* and the letter *u* by *oe*. The antiquated spelling of Jakarta as Djakarta is one such example. Likewise, names like Soekarno may also be spelt Sukarno. These tend to be viewed as interchangeable in the instance of personal names according to preference. However, the Dutch phonetics–influenced spellings were formally abandoned in 1950. Soerabaja became Surabaya, for example, pronounced precisely the same. In this book we tend to use the original spelling of given names like Soekarno or Soeharto but the modern spelling of place-names like Jakarta and

Surabaya. One often finds both spellings among person or brand-names in contemporary Indonesia and sometimes hybrids like Sur-jadjaja. The *u* is modern, while the *j* and *dj* are the antiquated *y* and *j*. This name is pronounced "sir ya jai yah," and even Indonesians stumble on it with "sir jah jah jah."

Mochtar is occasionally referred to in the historic literature by the spelling Muchtar (even by his nephew Abu Hanifah). This likely derives from confusion with the newer Indonesian phonetics post-1950. Hanifah assiduously applied modern phonetics in his writings, for example, spelling the Eijkman Institute as Eykman. We consider the spelling Mochtar definitive, as this is how he spelled his own name in his 1926 doctoral dissertation.

Many Javanese Indonesians have only one name, like Soekarno. Others have two names, the second of which may or may not be a surname. Mochtar is not Achmad Mochtar's surname. He didn't have one, just two given names. Some Indonesians do have surnames, and they are likely Eurocentric in heritage or they adopted a surname upon exposure to the western custom and the huge inconvenience of not being able to provide a surname to the myriad agencies demanding one. We make no effort to identify given versus actual surnames of the Indonesian players in the history conveyed in this book.

Reference in this history is made to the same city by three names: Jaya Karta, Batavia, and Jakarta. Another preceded all of these, Sunda Kelapa, but we dropped this detail from an already complex nomenclature. The city was referred to as Batavia until the eviction of the Dutch in 1942, when the liberated Indonesians renamed it Djakarta. However, the Dutch would successfully reclaim and hold the city as the colonial capital they still called Batavia between 1945 and 1949. The city finally became internationally acknowledged as Jakarta thereafter. In this history the city is referred to as Jakarta after the Dutch surrender to the Japanese in 1942.

Native speakers of English will recognize a few words of Indonesian/Malay language incorporated into their language. This is by no means a complete listing, but a few interesting and reasonably unequivocal examples. The word beriberi was likely introduced into the English language by the first known medical description of the illness in 1630 by Dutch physician Jacobus Bonitius, who encountered the illness on Java and referred to it by its locally known name. This was likely derived from a Sanskrit expression meaning, I cannot, or very weak. Orangutang derives from *orang hutan* or "man of the forest." To run "amok" means precisely that in Indonesia. Most Americans will recall schooldays when boys complained that by merely touching them, girls could give them "cooties"—some invisible infectious thing that somehow victimized boys by turning them more girl-like. In Indonesian, *kudis* is the word for scabies, a contagious skin infection by mites invisible to the naked eye. Its pronunciation is "koodies."

NOTES

1. Calamity

1. Theodore Friend, *The Blue-Eyed Enemy: Japan against the West in Java and Luzon, 1942–1945* (Princeton: Princeton University Press, 1988), 77.

2. Peter Post, William H. Frederick, Iris Heidebrink, and Shigeru Sato, eds., *The Encyclopedia of Indonesia in the Pacific War* (Boston: Brill, 2010), 197–212.

3. William A. Henderson, *From China, Burma, India to the Kwai* (Leon Junction TX: O & B, 1991), 82.

4. Robert Hardie, *The Burma-Siam Railway: The Secret Diary of Dr. Robert Hardie, 1942–1945* (London: Quadrant and the Imperial War Museum, 1983), 102.

5. E. E. Dunlop, *The War Diaries of Weary Dunlop: Java and the Burma-Thailand Railway, 1942–1945* (Ringwood VIC: Penguin, 1989), 264.

6. http://en.wikipedia.org/wiki/West_Kalimantan.

7. Friend, *Blue-Eyed Enemy*, 279.

8. http://en.wikipedia.org/wiki/Controversies_surrounding_Yasukuni_Shrine.

9. http://en.wikipedia.org/wiki/List_of_war_apology_statements_issued_by_Japan.

10. http://www.yasukuni.or.jp/english/about/deities.html.

11. http://japan.usembassy.gov/e/p/tp-20131226–01.html.

12. Post et al., *Encyclopedia of Indonesia in the Pacific War*, 403–20.

13. Exhibit 20, March 3, 1951, National Archives of Australia, series A471, item 81968, War Crimes—Military Tribunal—Nakamura Hirosato, barcode 720962.

14. Hal Gold, *Unit 731 Testimony* (North Clarendon VT: Tuttle, 2004).

2. Politics and Science

1. CDC, "The Association of Selected Cancers with Service in the U.S. Military in Vietnam," *Archives of Internal Medicine 150* (1990): 2473–2505; and N. A. Dalager, H. K. Kang, V. L. Burt, and L. Weatherbee, "Non-Hodgkins Lymphoma among Vietnam Veterans," *Journal of Occupational Medicine 33* (1991): 774–79.

2. http://en.wikipedia.org/wiki/Agent_Orange.

3. Friend, *Blue-Eyed Enemy*, 191.

4. Cindy Adams, *Sukarno: An Autobiography, as Told to Cindy Adams* (Indianapolis: Bobbs-Merrill, 1965), 193–94; Barbara Gifford Shimer, Guy Hobbs, and Theodore Friend, *Kenpeitai in Java and Sumatra: Selections from Nihon Kenpei Seishi* (Ithaca NY: Cornell University Southeast Asia Program Publications, 1986).

5. Post et al., *Encyclopedia of Indonesia in the Pacific War*, 197–212.

6. S. A. Weiss, "Prabowo Could Be Indonesia's Lee Kuan Yew," *Jakarta Post*, September 18, 2013; http://en.wikipedia.org/wiki/Indonesian_Democratic_Party—Struggle.

7. Ahdi Priamarizki, "Indonesian Election Sees Islamic Parties at a Crossroads," *Nation*, April 3, 2013.

3. Beginning of the End

1. Giles Milton, *Nathaniel's Nutmeg; or, The True Incredible Adventures of the Spice Trader Who Changed the Course of History* (London: Penguin, 2000).

2. Willard A. Hanna, *Bali Chronicles* (Hong Kong: Periplus, 2012).

3. Abu Hanifah, *Tales of a Revolution* (Sidney: Angus and Robertson, 1972), 106.

4. Winston Churchill, *The Second World War* (Boston: Mariner, 1986).

5. Shimer, Hobbs, and Friend, *Kenpeitai in Java and Sumatra*, 16.

6. Hanifah, *Tales of a Revolution*, 125.

7. Iris Chang, *The Rape of Nanking: The Forgotten History of World War II* (New York: Basic, 2012).

8. Iris Chang, suffering from psychotic depression, took her own life in 2004.

9. Edward Drea, Greg Bradsher, Robert Hanyok, James Lide, Michael Petersen, and Daqing Yang, *Researching Japanese War Crimes Records: Introductory Essays* (Washington DC: Nazi War Crimes and Japanese Imperial Government Records Interagency Working Group, 2006), 7.

10. Shimer, Hobbs, and Friend, *Kenpeitai in Java and Sumatra*, 27.

11. Post et al., *Encyclopedia of Indonesia in the Pacific War*, 148–60.

12. Shimer, Hobbs, and Friend, *Kenpeitai in Java and Sumatra*, 69.

13. Friend, *Blue-Eyed Enemy*, 108.

4. Netherlands East Indies

1. Friend, *Blue-Eyed Enemy*, 20.

2. Friend, *Blue-Eyed Enemy*, 20.

3. Friend, *Blue-Eyed Enemy*, 21.

4. Kenneth J. Carpenter, *Beriberi, White Rice, and Vitamin B: A Disease, a Cause, a Cure* (Berkeley: University of California Press, 2000).

5. David McCullough, *The Path between the Seas: The Creation of the Panama Canal, 1870–1914* (New York: Simon and Schuster, 1978).

6. Philip H. Manson-Bahr, *History of the School of Tropical Medicine in London, 1899–1949* (London: H. K. Lewis, 1956).

7. Maria J. Otten-van Stockum, "Rabies Research in the Netherlands Indies." *Mededeelingen van den Dienst der Volksgezondheid in Nederlandsch-Indie* 30 (1941): 269–79.

5. Coming of Age

1. Friend, *Blue-Eyed Enemy*, 24.

2. Friend, *Blue-Eyed Enemy*, 23.

3. That language had been a lingua franca of trade in the Indonesian and Philippine Archipelagos and the Malay Peninsula for centuries, originating from the powerful Hindu Srivijaya dynasty of Sumatra around 900 AD. It is the basis of modern Indonesian, Malaysian, and Tagalog (of the Philippines) languages.

4. Indonesian language before 1950 applied Dutch phonetics in spelling that was then formally abandoned. Thus the name Tjipto Mangoengkoesoemo became Cipto Mangungkusumo. The *c* and *tj* of Indonesian and Dutch phonetics, respectively, is each pronounced as the *ch* of English phonetics. Throughout this book we strive to maintain period-specific phonetics in spelling, as with Boedi Oetomo (Budi Utomo in modern spelling), but we do not do so for place-names, like Djakarta and Soerabaja (Jakarta and Surabaya).

5. Moh. Ali Hanafiah, *Drama Kedokteran Terbesar* (Jakarta: Yayasan Gedung-Gedung Bersejarah, 1976), 60–61.

6. http://www.youtube.com/watch?v=Icil_VRnPUw.

7. Adams, *Sukarno*, 194.

8. O. E. Engelen, A. B. Loebis, F. Pattiasina, A. Ciptoprawiro, S. Joedodibroto, Oetarjo, and I. Siregar, *Lahirnya Satu Bangsa dan Negara* (Jakarta: University of Indonesia Press, 1987), 25–27.

9. Sarwono Prawirohardjo, "Pendidikan dokter dalam masa pendudukan Jepang dan dalam masa perjuang kemerdekaan fisik," in *125 Tahun Pendidikan Dokter di Indonesia: 1851–1976* (Jakarta: Ikatan Dokter Indonesia, 1976), 35–39.

6. Excellence

1. Jan Peter Verhave, *The Moses of Malaria: Nicolaas H. Swellengrebel (1885–1970) Abroad and at Home* (Rotterdam: Erasmus University Press, 2011).

2. W.A.P. Schüffner, "Two Subjects Relating to the Epidemiology of Malaria." *Journal of the Malaria Institute of India* 1 (1938): 221–56.

3. W. J. Terpstra, "Historical Perspectives in Leptospirosis," *Indian Journal of Medical Microbiology* 24 (2006): 316–20.

4. It is Japanese custom to write the surname first, followed by the given name. Throughout this book we follow that format for all of the Japanese names except Hideyo Noguchi and Shibasabura Kitazato in the previous chapter. As many Japanese and Koreans who live and work in the West do, they formatted name order to accommodate western custom, probably to avoid confusion and real nuisance; Noguchi Hideyo became presented as Hideyo Noguchi, by which he is most widely known.

5. H. Noguchi, "*Leptospira icteroides* and Yellow Fever," *Proceedings of the National Academy of Sciences* (1919): 111.

6. M. Theiler and A. W. Sellards, "The Relationship of *L. icterohaemorrhagiae*

and *L. icteroides* as Determined by the Pfeiffer Phenomenon in Guinea Pigs," *American Journal of Tropical Medicine* 6 (1927): 383–402.

7. B. M. van Driel and Achmad Mochtar, "Oderzoekingen amtrent eenige leptospiren-stammen," *Geneeskundig Tijdschrift voor Nederlandsch-Indie* 67 (1927): 763–65.

8. John Farley, *To Cast Out Disease: A History of the International Health Division of the Rockefeller Foundation (1913–1951)* (New York: Oxford University Press, 2004).

9. Isabel R. Plesset, *Noguchi and His Patrons* (Rutherford NJ: Fairleigh Dickinson University Press, 1980), 249.

10. A. Stokes, J. H. Bauer, and N. P. Hudson, "The Transmission of Yellow fever to Macacus Rhesus," *Journal of the American Medical Association* 96 (1928): 253–54.

11. Plesset, *Noguchi and His Patrons*, 255.

12. Simon Flexner, "Hideyo Noguchi: A Biographical Sketch," *Science*, June 28, 1929, 653–60.

13. J. F. Schacher, review of *Noguchi and His Patrons* in *American Journal of Tropical Medicine and Hygiene* 30 (1981): 296–97.

14. Mochtar, *Onderzoekingen Omtrent Eenige Leptospiren-stammen* (Amsterdam: Universiteits Boekhandel Grimburgwal 11, 1927).

15. Hanifah, *Tales of a Revolution*, 127.

7. New Reality

1. Hanifah, *Tales of a Revolution*, 179.

2. Hanifah, *Tales of a Revolution*, 179–81.

3. Friend, *Blue-Eyed Enemy*, 196.

4. Friend, *Blue-Eyed Enemy*, 106.

5. Post et al., *Encyclopedia of Indonesia in the Pacific War*, 71–86.

6. "Dari 'Non-Cooperation' ke Cooperation," *Panji Pustaka*, September 5, 1942, 4.

7. Moh. Ali Hanafiah, Bahder Djohan, and S. Surono, 125th Pendidikan Dokter di Indonesia, 1851–1976 (Jakarta: Panitya Peringatan, 1976).

8. Hanafiah, *Drama Kedokteran Terbesar*, 60.

9. Hanifah, *Tales of a Revolution*, 124.

10. Post et al., *Encyclopedia of Indonesia in the Pacific War*, 212–17.

11. Pans Schomper, *Chaos after Paradise: The Promise of the Japanese Egg Man*, translated from Dutch by Greta Kwik (Amsterdam: Dorned, 1995).

8. Klender

1. Post et al., *Encyclopedia of Indonesia in the Pacific War*, 197–218.

2. Sutanto Atmosumarto, *A Learner's Comprehensive Dictionary of Indonesian* (London: Atma Stanton, 2004).

3. Post et al., *Encyclopedia of Indonesia in the Pacific War*, 22–24.

4. Willem Wanrooy, "The Will to Live," http://members.iinet.net.au/~vanderkp /wiltoliv.html.

5. Friend, *Blue-Eyed Enemy*, 83.

6. Hanifah, *Tales of a Revolution*, 122.

7. Hanifah, *Tales of a Revolution*, 139.

8. Post et al., *Encyclopedia of Indonesia in the Pacific War*, 184–97.

9. W. E. Johns and R. A. Kelly, *No Surrender: The Story of William E. Johns, DSM, Chief Ordnance Artificer, and How He Survived after the Sinking of the HMS Exeter in the Java Sea in March 1942* (London: George G. Harrap, 1969), 136.

10. Post et al., *Encyclopedia of Indonesia in the Pacific War*, 197–201.

11. Harry A. Poeze, "The Road to Hell: The Construction of a Railway Line in West Java during the Japanese Occupation," in *Asian Labor in the Wartime Japanese Empire*, ed. P. H. Kratoska (Singapore: National University of Singapore Press, 2009), 162.

12. Poeze, "Road to Hell." 163.

13. Adams, *Sukarno*, 123.

14. Post et al., *Encyclopedia of Indonesia in the Pacific War*, 197–218.

15. Adams, *Sukarno*, 194.

16. Adams, *Sukarno*, 184–86.

17. Post et al., *Encyclopedia of Indonesia in the Pacific War*, 197–218.

18. Hanifah, *Tales of a Revolution*, 122.

19. Post et al., *Encyclopedia of Indonesia in the Pacific War*, 197–218.

20. Hanafiah, *Drama Kedokteran Terbesar*.

21. Friend, *Blue-Eyed Enemy*, 193–96.

22. H. Amura, *Bahder Djohan: Pengabdi Kemanusiaan* (Jakarta: Gunung Agung, 1980).

9. Darkness

1. In the original Indonesian language testimony, Jatman alternatively refers to Mochtar by the honorific "Prof." or "Pak." Literally translated "Pak" means "Mister," but in Indonesia "Pak" is equally honorific.

2. Friend, *Blue-Eyed Enemy*, 195.

10. Tetanus

1. P. van Leersum, "Chapters in the History of Cinchona. III. Junghuhn and Cinchona Cultivation," in *Science and Scientists in the Netherlands Indies*, ed. P. Honig and F. Verdoorn, 190–96.

2. "Meninjau Kesehatan Rakjat," *Pandji Poestaka*, March 8, 1943.

3. Post et al., *Encyclopedia of Indonesia in the Pacific War*, 417–19.

4. A. P. Long, "Tetanus Toxoid: Its Use in the United States Army," *American Journal of Public Health* 33 (1943): 53–57.

5. A. J. Fulthorpe, "Estimation of Tetanus Toxoid by Different Methods, Including Haemagglutination Inhibition," *Immunology* 1 (October 1958): 365–72.

11. Modus Operandi

1. Post et al., *Encyclopedia of Indonesia in the Pacific War*, 148–60.

2. Friend, *Blue-Eyed Enemy*, 196.

3. Friend, *Blue-Eyed Enemy*, 196–97.

4. Greg Bradsher, "The Exploitation of Captured and Seized Japanese Records Relating to War Crimes, 1942–1945," in *Researching Japanese War Crimes Records: Introductory Essays*, ed. Edward Drea et al. (Washington DC: Nazi War Crimes and Japanese Imperial Government Records Interagency Working Group, 2006).

5. Drea et al., *Researching Japanese War Crimes Records*, 9.

6. National Archives of Australia, Series A471, Item 81968, War Crimes—Military Tribunal—NAKAMURA Hirosato.

7. Neil Z. Miller, *Vaccines: Are They Really Safe and Effective?* Santa Fe: New Atlantean, 2002.

8. Hanafiah, *Drama Kedokteran Terbesar*, 63.

9. W. U. Eckart, "Malaria and World War II: German Malaria Experiments, 1939–1945," *Parasitologia* 42 (2000): 53–58.

10. Hanifah, *Tales of a Revolution*, 127.

11. Thanks are due to Captain Trevor R. Jones, at the time (2010) commanding officer of the U.S. Naval Medical Research Unit No. 2 in Jakarta, for recognizing the poem and pointing this out to us.

12. Legacy

1. *Bapak* means "father," but is also used honorifically, as it was in this instance. Bahar was not Ayal's son but an employee and resident of his home.

2. Hanifah, *Tales of a Revolution*, 333–34.

3. Adams, *Sukarno*, 193–94

4. Hanifah, *Tales of a Revolution*, 127–28.

Epilogue

1. Moh. Ali Hanafiah, *77 Tahun Riwayat Hidup* (Jakarta: privately published, 1977), 82–83.

2. Thanks due to G. Michael Baird, brother of JKB and a lawman, who offered this very useful and illustrative analogy.

3. Post et al., *Encyclopedia of Indonesia in the Pacific War*, 419.

4. Quotation cited in Drea et al., *Researching Japanese War Crimes Records*, 7.

SELECTED BIBLIOGRAPHY

Political and Military History of the Pacific War

Atmosumarto, Sutanto. *A Learner's Comprehensive Dictionary of Indonesian*. London: Atma Stanton, 2004.

Cox, Jeffrey R. *Rising Sun, Falling Skies: The Disastrous Java Sea Campaign of World War II*. New York: Osprey, 2014.

Daws, Gavan. *Prisoners of the Japanese: POWs of World War II in the Pacific*. New York: William Morrow, 1996.

Hornfischer, James D. *Ship of Ghosts: The Story of the USS Houston, FDR's Legendary Lost Cruiser, and the Epic Saga of Her Survivors*. New York: Bantam, 2006.

Johns, W. E., and R. A. Kelly. *No Surrender: The Story of William E. Johns, DSM, Chief Ordnance Artificer, and How He Survived after the Sinking of the HMS Exeter in the Java Sea in March 1942*. London: George G. Harrap, 1969.

Smith, Colin. *Singapore Burning: Heroism and Surrender in World War II*. New York: Viking, 2005.

Toland, John. *The Rising Sun: The Decline and Fall of the Japanese Empire, 1936–1945*. New York: Random House, 1970; reprint, New York: Modern Library, 2003.

Van der Vat, Dan. *Pacific Campaign: The U.S.–Japanese Naval War, 1941–1945*. New York: Simon & Schuster, 1992.

Japanese Occupation of Indonesia

Friend, Theodore. *The Blue-Eyed Enemy: Japan against the West in Java and Luzon, 1942–1945*. Princeton: Princeton University Press, 1988.

Gin, Ooi Keat. *The Japanese Occupation of Borneo, 1941–1945*. Routledge Studies in the Modern History of Asia. New York: Routledge, 2011.

Hovinga, Henk. *The Sumatra Railroad: Final Destination Pakan Baroe, 1943–1945*. Translated by Robert Rouveroy. Leiden: KITLV Press, 2010.

Post, Peter, William H. Frederick, Iris Heidebrink, and Shigeru Sato, eds. *The Encyclopedia of Indonesia in the Pacific War*. Boston: Brill, 2010.

Ockerse, Ralph, and Evelijn Blaney. *Our Childhood in the Former Colonial Dutch East Indies: Recollections before and during Our Wartime Internment by the Japanese.* Bloomington: Xlibris, 2011.

Sato, Shigeru. *War, Nationalism, and Peasants: Java under the Japanese Occupation, 1942–1945.* Armonk NY: M. E. Sharpe, 1997.

Schomper, Pans. *Chaos after Paradise: The Promise of the Japanese Egg Man.* Translated from Dutch by Greta Kwik. Amsterdam: Dorned, 1995.

Shimer, Barbara Gifford, Guy Hobbs, and Theodore Friend. *The Kenpeitai in Java and Sumatra: Selections from Nihon Kenpei Seishi.* Ithaca: Cornell University Southeast Asia Program Publications, 1986.

History of Netherlands East Indies and Indonesia

Jong, L. de. *The Collapse of a Colonial Society: The Dutch in Indonesia during the Second World War.* Leiden : KITLV Press, 2002.

Gouda, Frances, and Thijs Brocades Zaalberg. *American Visions of the Netherlands East Indies/Indonesia: U.S. Foreign Policy and Indonesian Nationalism, 1920–1949.* Amsterdam: Amsterdam University Press, 2003.

Taylor, Jean Gelman. *Indonesia: Peoples and Histories.* New Haven: Yale University Press, 2004.

Hanifah, Abu. *Tales of a Revolution.* Sidney: Angus and Robertson, 1972.

Mann, Richard. *400 Years and More of the British in Indonesia.* 2nd ed. Privately published, 2013.

McMahon, Robert J. *Colonialism and Cold War: The United States and the Struggle for Indonesian Independence, 1945–1949.* Ithaca: Cornell University Press, 1981.

Milton, Giles. *Nathaniel's Nutmeg; or, The True and Incredible Adventures of the Spice Trader Who Changed the Course of History.* London: Penguin Books, 2000.

Pisani, Elizabeth. *Indonesia Etc.: Exploring the Improbable Nation.* New York: W. W. Norton, 2014.

Ricklefs, M. C. *A History of Modern Indonesia since c. 1200.* 4th ed. Stanford: Stanford University Press.

Tantri, K'tut. *Revolt in Paradise: One Woman's Fight for Freedom in Indonesia.* New York: Potter, 1989.

Winchester, Simon. *Krakatoa: The Day the World Exploded, August 27, 1883.* New York: Harper Perennial, 2005.

Colonialism and Medicine

Anderson, Warwick. *Colonial Pathologies: American Tropical Medicine, Race, and Hygiene in the Philippines.* Durham: Duke University Press, 2006. 368pp.

Bashford, Alison. *Imperial Hygiene: A Critical History of Colonialism, Nationalism, and Public Health.* New York: Palgrave Macmillan, 2014. 280pp.

Johnson, Ryan. *Tropical Medicine and Imperial Power: Science, Hygiene, and Health in the Late British Empire.* International Library of Colonial History. London: I. B. Tauris, 2014. 320pp.

Harrison, Mark. *Medicine in an Age of Commerce and Empire: Britain and Its Tropical Colonies, 1660–1830*. New York: Oxford University Press, 2010. 384pp.

Neill, Deborah. *Networks in Tropical Medicine: Internationalism, Colonialism, and the Rise of a Medical Specialty, 1890–1930*. Stanford: Stanford University Press, 2012. 312pp.

Relevant Medical History

Carpenter, Kenneth J. *Beriberi, White Rice, and Vitamin B: A Disease, a Cause, a Cure*. Berkeley: University of California Press, 2000.

Farley, John. *To Cast Out Disease: A History of the International Health Division of the Rockefeller Foundation (1913–1951)*. New York: Oxford University Press, 2004.

Kita, Atsushi. *Dr. Noguchi's Journey: A Life of Medical Search and Discovery*. Translated by Peter Durfee. New York: Kodansha, 2003.

Plesset, Isabel R. *Noguchi and His Patrons*. Rutherford NJ: Fairleigh Dickinson University Press, 1980.

Rocco, Fiammetta. *Quinine: Malaria and the Quest for a Cure That Changed the World*. New York: Harper Perennial, 2004.

Verhave, Jan Peter. *The Moses of Malaria: Nicolaas H. Swellengrebel (1885–1970) Abroad and at Home*. Rotterdam: Erasmus University Press, 2011.

Japanese Atrocities during the Pacific War

Barenblatt, Daniel. *A Plague upon Humanity: The Hidden History of Japan's Biological Warfare Program*. New York: Harper Perennial, 2005.

Chang, Iris. *The Rape of Nanking: The Forgotten Holocaust of World War II*. New York: Basic Books, 2012.

Gold, Hal. *Unit 731 Testimony*. North Clarendon VT: Tuttle, 2004.

Krotoska, Paul H., ed. *Asian Labor in the Wartime Japanese Empire: Unknown Histories*. Armonk NY: M. E. Sharpe, 2005.

Li, Peter, ed. *Japanese War Crimes*. New Brunswick: Transaction, 2003.

Nie, Jing Bao, Nanyan Guo, Mark Selden, and Arthur Kleinman, eds. *Japan's Wartime Medical Atrocities: Comparative Inquiries in Science, History, and Ethics*. Asia's Transformations series. New York: Routledge, 2011.

Rees, Laurence. *Horror in the East: Japan and the Atrocities of World War II*. Cambridge: Da Capo Press, 2002.

Tanaka, Yuki. *Hidden Horrors: Japanese War Crimes in World War II*. Boulder: Westview Press, 1997.

Williams, Peter, and David Wallace. *Unit 731: Japan's Secret Biological Warfare in World War II*. New York: Free Press, 1989.

Japanese War Tribunals

Drea, Edward, Greg Bradsher, Robert Hanyok, James Lide, Michael Petersen, and Daqing Yang. *Researching Japanese War Crimes Records: Introductory Essays*.

Washington DC: Nazi War Crimes and Japanese Imperial Government Records Interagency Working Group, 2006.

Maga, Tim. *Judgment at Tokyo: The Japanese War Crimes Trials*. Lexington: University of Kentucky Press, 2001.

Piccagallo, Philip R. *The Japanese on Trial: Allied War Crimes Operations in the East, 1945–1951*. Austin: University of Texas Press, 1980.

Nazi Medical Atrocities and Justice

Greene, Joshua. *Justice at Dachau: The Trials of an American Prosecutor*. New York: Broadway Books, 2003.

Kulish, Nicholas. *The Eternal Nazi: From Mauthausen to Cairo, the Relentless Pursuit of SS Doctor Aribert Heim*. New York: Doubleday, 2014.

Schmidt, Ulf. *Justice at Nuremburg: Leo Alexander and the Nazi Doctors' Trial*. St. Antony's series. 2nd ed. New York: Palgrave Macmillan, 2006. 386pp.

Schmidt, Ulf. *Karl Brandt the Nazi Doctor: Medicine and Power in the Third Reich*. London: Bloomsbury Academic, 2008.

Weindling, Paul Julian. *Nazi Medicine and the Nuremburg Trials: From Medical War Crimes to Informed Consent*. New York: Palgrave Macmillan, 2006.

Contemporary East Asian Geopolitics

Economy, Elizabeth, and Michael Levi. *By All Means Necessary: How China's Resource Quest Is Changing the World*. New York: Oxford University Press, 2014.

Goh, Evelyn. *The Struggle for Order: Hegemony, Hierarchy, and Transition in Post–Cold War East Asia*. New York: Oxford University Press, 2013.

Kaplan, Robert D. *Asia's Cauldron: The South China Sea and the End of a Stable Pacific*. New York: Random House, 2014.

Lind, Jennifer. *Sorry States: Apologies in International Politics*. Cornell Studies in Security Affairs. Ithaca: Cornell University Press, 2010.

Slater, Dan. *Ordering Power: Contentious Politics and Authoritarian Leviathans in Southeast Asia*. New York: Cambridge University Press, 2010.

INDEX

China (*cont.*)
Japanese war crimes in, xii, 46–47; and Japanese war responsibility denial, 12, 13–14, 248–49; U.S. policy and, 15, 247
Cho Konosuke, 193
Christians, 31
Churchill, Winston, 39, 40
Cimahi cemetery, F31, 129–30, 233–34
Cipto Hospital, 77, 141
Collier, W. A., 99
colonialism: East Indies history of, 53–55; effort to reform, 55–56; as Japanese desire, 4, 26–27, 103, 106, 250; legacy of, 249–50; Pacific War destruction of, 102–3, 222–24, 244–45; Southeast Asia history of, 10–11. *See also* Dutch colonialism
"Comfort Women," 128
communists, 25–26, 111
Confucianists, 31
Coral Sea, Battle of (1942), 122
Cruz, Ozwaldo, 60

Darling, S. T., 59
Darul Islam insurgency, 112
De Haan, Johannes, 62
de Reede, C. A., 99
Descombey, P., 182
Dewantoro, Ki Hadjar, 80, 105, 109, 195
Dinger, Professor, 155, 234
Diponegoro, Achmad, 113
diptheria, 181–82
Djoehana, R. M., 99
Djoehana Wiradikarta, 221; imprisonment of, 154, 160, 168–69, 176
Djohan, Bahder, 141–42, 144, 153
Djohan, Baheer, 99
Djumina, 131–32
Donath, W. P., 58
Drama Kedokteran Terbesar (Hanafiah), 33, 152, 168, 236
Dutch colonialism, 53–69; attempted restoration of, 48, 245; British defense of, 220; history of, 2, 37, 53–54; Japanese shattering of, 28, 37–38, 42–

43, 102–3, 105; police force used by, 53, 102; propaganda against nationalists by, 113; reform of, 55–56; war of independence against, 27, 81, 111, 112, 219–21, 223, 234. *See also* Netherlands East Indies
Dutch East Indies Company, 2, 37

East Timor, 223, 224
education, colonial, 73–75
Eijkman, Christiaan, F4, 80; and beriberi, 57–59; Nobel Prize awarded to, 56, 59, 228–29
Eijkman Institute: bacteriology laboratory in, F5; as beacon of racial and social justice, 65; buildings of, F3, 229–31; closing of (1965), 225, 226; decline and death of, xvi, 219, 221; establishment of, 60; under Japanese occupation, 80, 116, 117, 120–21; and Klender events, 142, 144–45, 148, 149–52, 172, 226; Mochtar joining staff of, 99; Mochtar memorial ceremony at, 240–42; native Indonesian scientists at, xiii, 61, 65; rebirth of, 227–30; staff of, F21, F22, 65; work on tropical medicine by, xiii, 57–58, 60–63
Ekawati, Lenny, 131
empat serangkai, 80, 107, 151, 195; and Japanese occupation system, 105–6
Encyclopedia of Indonesia in the Pacific War, 139, 140, 153
Esseveld, H., 99
Eurasians, 16–17, 47, 117–19

Flexner, Simon, 88, 90, 93, 95, 218
Flu, P. C., 59
Foundation for Historic Buildings in Jakarta, 152
Friend, Theodore: on Dutch East Indies, 55, 74–75; on Japanese rule, 11–12, 45; on Mochtar affair, 141, 153, 195
Fulthorpe, A. J., 191

Gerindra, 30
Gin, Ooi Keat, 107, 114, 115

Islam, 72–73
Islamists, 30, 31, 111–12
Israel, 248

Jakarta: historical names for, 2, 253; population of, 139. *See also* Batavia
Jansen, B. C. P., 58
Japan (contemporary): demands for truthful accounting by, xvii, 13–14, 128; honoring of war criminals in, 12–13, 18, 36, 46; nationalism in, xiii, 247–48; refusal to acknowledge war crimes by, xvii–xviii, 13, 15, 36, 248–50; tributes to Japanese war effort in, 24, 245, 247–48; U.S. relationship with, 14, 246–47
Japan (militarist): Asian conquests by, 38–43; bombing of Pearl Harbor by, 35, 38; bushido creed in, 49; colonial empire sought by, 4, 26–27, 103, 106, 250; defeats in Pacific War, 48–49, 107, 110, 122–25, 196; fascist worldview of, 4, 36; motivations for Pacific War by, 17–18; propaganda about Asia by, 11, 104; racism of, 4, 11–12, 50; sexual enslavement employed by, 128, 132–33
Japanese Journal of Veterinary Medicine, 99
Japanese occupation of Indonesia: army-navy conflict under, 198–99; of Batavia, 42, 101, 116; of Borneo, 42, 106–7, 114, 115; colonialist functioning of, 103, 106–7; Dutch colonialism shattered by, 28, 37–38, 42–43, 102–3, 105; Dutch colonists under, 16–17, 116–17, 117–18; Eijkman Institute under, 80, 116, 117, 120–21; Eurasians under, 16–17, 47, 117–19; Indonesian independence maneuvers by, 107, 110, 113; Indonesian nationalists and, 25–27, 103, 104, 105–6; initial welcoming of, 25, 102, 105; instances of humane treatment by, 119–20, 167; Japanese civilian intellectuals in, 103–4, 119–20; and Joyoboyo prophecy, 3, 25; martial law imposed by, 103; murder

of intellectuals under, 45, 113–14, 115; physicians under, 45, 113–14, 115–16; plots and conspiracies fabricated by, 7, 16, 114–15, 151–52; political system established by, 105–6, 119, 194–95; propaganda by, 49, 104, 131, 135, 136, 186; recruitment of romusha by, 4–5, 28, 131–32, 136, 137–38, 140; romusha holocaust under, 4–7, 127–29, 135–36; seizure of wealth under, 114–15; sexual enslavement under, 132–33; Soekarno and, 26–27, 47, 79–80, 105, 106, 107–10, 111, 132, 137, 151; of Sumatra, 42, 115, 130, 193, 198; summary executions by, 5, 7, 15–16, 44–45, 117, 122, 128; takeover of Dutch East Indies, 42–43; treatment of POWs by, 6, 10–11, 133–34
Jatman, Mr., 61, 234; imprisonment of, 154, 169–72, 175–76; and Klender events, 144–45, 149, 165
Java, 42, 115, 193; history of, 1, 53–54; romusha in, 134–35, 136
Joedo, Wisnoe, 61, 65
Johns, William E., 133–34
Joyoboyo, 1; prophecies of, 2, 3, 100, 109, 123
Junghuhn, Franz Wilhelm, 180
Jun Yoshio, 114
Junyu Maru sinking, 129–30
Juzar, Taty Delma, 115, 161, 241; photos of, F14, F40, 66–68

Kadiroen, 61
Kenpeitai: about, 43–48; arrests in Klender case by, 151; Eurasians as target of, 118; executions by, 44–46, 47–48; executions of after war, 193–94; instances of humane treatment by, 166–67; interrogation of Indonesian scholars by, 3; Jakarta headquarters of, 156–57, F26; management of Klender investigation by, 50–51, 187; poster of agents from, F28; Tokkeitai as Indonesian partners to, 161; torture and interrogations by, 33, 141, 156–57, 158–59, 160, 162–66, 173,

CPSIA information can be obtained
at www.ICGtesting.com
Printed in the USA
LVOW11*1550291117
558023LV00007B/73/P